CANCER AND LEUKAEMIA

Jan de Vries was born in Holland in 1937 and grew up in occupied territory during the difficult war years. Graduating in pharmacy, he turned to alternative medicine. His most influential teacher was Alfred Vogel in Switzerland, and they have worked together closely for 35 years.

In 1980 he and his family moved to Scotland and settled in Troon, where he set up a residential clinic. He also has clinics in Edinburgh, Ireland, the Republic of Ireland and London. He lectures throughout the world and is a regular broadcaster on BBC radio.

D0791785

Books available from the same author

By Appointment Only series

Arthritis, Rheumatism and Psoriasis (second edition)
Asthma and Bronchitis
Heart and Blood Circulatory Problems
Migraine and Epilepsy (fourth impression)
The Miracle of Life
Multiple Sclerosis (second edition)
Neck and Back Problems (second edition)
Realistic Weight Control (second edition)
Skin Diseases
Stomach and Bowel Disorders
Stress and Nervous Disorders (second edition, second impression)
Traditional Home and Herbal Remedies (second edition)
Viruses, Allergies and the Immune System (fourth impression)
Who's Next? (second edition)

Nature's Gift series

Body Energy
Food
Water - Healer or Poison?

Well Woman series

Menopause
Menstrual and Pre-menstrual Tension

The Jan de Vries Healthcare series

Questions and Answers on Family Health
Life Without Arthritis - the Maori Way

Jan de Vries

Cancer and Leukaemia
An alternative approach

By Appointment Only series

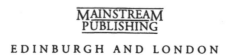

MAINSTREAM
PUBLISHING

EDINBURGH AND LONDON

First published in Great Britain in 1988 by
MAINSTREAM PUBLISHING COMPANY
(EDINBURGH) LTD
7 Albany Street
Edinburgh EH1 3UG

ISBN 1 84018 555 4

This edition, 2001
Reprinted 2003

A catalogue record for this book is available
from the British Library

Typeset in Palatino
Printed and bound in Great Britain by
Antony Rowe Ltd, Chippenham, Wiltshire

Contents

This book is dedicated to
the Jan de Vries Benevolent Trust
which was founded
for the benefit of patients in need.

Registered Office:
18 Bristo Place,
Edinburgh.

Jacket illustration: *Petasites officinalis*

Foreword

I HAD THE great fortune and privilege to meet Dr Jan de Vries a good number of years ago at a Cancer Convention for lay people in Los Angeles, California, USA. I very much enjoyed his talks and found out that we shared the same philosophy concerning the treatment of chronic diseases, especially cancer. So, a wonderful friendship was immediately started.

He graciously invited me to visit his place and be his guest for as long as I could stay. I gladly accepted and a couple of years later I flew with my wife to Scotland and went to his beautiful clinic. We stayed there for a whole week in the special guest suite and were royally treated.

I was really impressed with the numerous patients who arrived continually (by appointment only) to be treated for all kinds of problems; also at the happy atmosphere and the successful results the patients reported. His programmes, I could witness, were based exclusively on non-aggressive natural procedures, helped by wonderful psychological and spiritual advice, given in a completely natural and gifted way. I realised that I was watching the medical practice of a *true physician*, and I thanked God for that.

Now my dear friend has asked me to write the foreword to his latest book in the *By Appointment Only* series, dealing with cancer. Although I know I am not the most qualified person to do him justice, I gladly accepted his invitation.

I bet that many people, when they see the notice about the publication of this book, will make the usual comment: "Another book about cancer for the lay person? Are there not plenty of good books already?"

My answer is a straight *no*. There are *not* enough books about this controversial subject. Cancer is such a complex issue, with so many unsolved problems remaining in the areas of general management, success rates and prevention, that the reader will find this book to be an important source of knowledge greatly needed for the general public and even for open-minded health practitioners.

Fifty years of intense cancer research by the most qualified scientists all around the world, having at their disposal the most modern equipment, luxurious facilities and practically unlimited amounts of money, have not yielded the fruits so eagerly expected.

Early in 1970 the National Cancer Institute of the United States of America declared their "War against Cancer", with the firm conviction that in ten years they would have the solution to the problem. However, early in 1980 they had to accept that only a few types of cancer had been conquered. They tried to maintain optimism through several publications during the next five years. But in May 1986 that optimism received a tremendous blow when Drs Bailar III and Smith, from the Public Health School of Harvard, published a paper in the *New England Journal of Medicine* about their research on the progress in cancer treatment during the last thirty-two years. According to their conclusions, present cancer treatments should be considered a "qualified failure", because the fruits are very little in comparison with the time, effort and expenditure spent over so many years. "What has been wrong in the research?" they wondered. Then they urged the scientists to re-evaluate their programmes and seek out more realistic approaches, giving due attention to the preventive programmes which had been neglected for so long.

8

One of the many reasons why progress has been so desperately slow, is that throughout this century medical practice has been orientated towards strictly scientific grounds, to the point that modern oncologists affirm that cancer should be approached using only the Biomedical Model. This is obviously wrong. The human being is not just a biological subject. It is a trinity. To artificially separate the physical body from the soul and the spirit has been a great mistake. Modern science, being totally agnostic, has not proved itself to be the ultimate weapon with which to fight human illness. Medicine is, and always will, be a combination of *art* and *science*.

Jesus of Nazareth, the greatest physician of all times, treated his patients to make them whole again, that is, healing the body, the mind and the spirit simultaneously. Later on Hippocrates, Galen, Paracelsus and many others treated their patients in the same way.

In this century, especially during the last twenty-five years, many physicians have tried to go back to the original approach, being unhappy about the materialistic and excessively aggressive cancer treatments used by the highly scientifically trained oncologists. Those physicians have been attacked and even persecuted for their unorthodox views and called by the worst adjectives. But the results they are obtaining make perseverance worth while!

Not long ago, a doctor with great experience in cancer research and treatments reluctantly accepted the invitation of a mutual friend to visit my institution and learn the truth about my work. He came with the intention of making a very short, polite visit; but he stayed for almost two hours! It was the most exciting exchange of ideas I have ever had with a pure scientist and at the end he gave me the best illustration I have heard of what he believed the problem of conquering cancer to be.

He likened cancer to a giant puzzle with millions of small, bizarre pieces to accommodate in order to solve the problem. Scientific research, through the years, has been able to put together thousands of pieces starting from one side of the

9

puzzle where the most difficult pieces should be put in place through the co-operation of all interested parties.

Dr Jan de Vries belongs to the group of visionary, non-conventional physicians who have been able to correctly accommodate many of the pieces in the puzzle, having started at the opposite side from where the pure scientists are working. He uses common sense, intuition, natural methods, psychology and spiritual help in a balanced way, in addition to drawing on his scientific background. His approach is both realistic and effective, combining medicines with positive thinking, hope, faith and love. Science and Art.

This is why I assure the reader that Dr Jan de Vries' book is not just another commonplace publication about cancer or a mere compilation of what many others have written.

Jan is sharing with the world his own unique experience of many years of successful medical practice, which I am sure will be of great benefit for millions of potential patients who can learn how to prevent cancer. This book is a blessing to those who, unfortunately, are already victims of this terrible illness, bringing a new ray of hope to their shattered lives.

Dr Ernesto Contreras R MD

1

What is Cancer?

CANCER! How often have we witnessed the terror the very sound of this word strikes in today's society? Cancer does not respect status and will attack the rich and the poor, the old as well as the young.

I was still very young when I first became aware of this most dreaded disease. My younger sister was born during the winter of 1944-45, which in the Netherlands, where I originate from, is commonly referred to as the "Hungerwinter", for obvious reasons. How well I remember that wintry, grim morning with death and destruction all around us. My mother — a very brave woman — was conducting a meeting which was interrupted by sirens warning us of an air raid and when the all-clear sounded she asked one of her friends to take me with her. The local doctor was informed and also the midwife.

Although still very young I realised that something unusual was going on when I was taken away by my mother's friend. The subsequent birth of my little sister seemed like a ray of sunshine and hope in a world full of misery and danger. It was something that cheered us all and to the adults it acted temporarily as a diversion from their worries about the war.

A day later I was back home again, once arrangements enough had been made for the people in hiding from the Germans for whom my mother had accepted responsibility. It was then that a scaly patch was noticed on the back of my newly born baby sister and the local doctor was asked for his opinion. He was not too happy about it and favoured a second opinion. He told Mother that he suspected it to be a kind of skin cancer. This sounded serious and yet it seemed so unbelievable to discover this in such a young baby.

Nowadays I seem to come across such problems so much more frequently and I am staggered to see this complaint so much on the increase. The devastating effects of cancer strike at the basics of the human body, namely the cells. We see only too often that the regenerative cells come under attack, which could be possibly due to dietary causes or an enzyme deficiency or imbalance. Insufficient vitamins and minerals could also be a contributory factor in that these cells are not allowed to function properly. We must never overlook the fact, too, that stress has a detrimental effect on our health.

Bearing this in mind, it was not so strange to hear, as I once did, an old professor relate in a lecture that every day on waking up, he wishes his cells a "Good morning!".

If I had my wish we would never see the stress of war repeated, and no doubt this goes for the majority of people who lived through those days. However, our present lives are by no means free of stress and to my thinking this could have a lot of bearing on the increasing incidence of cancer. But not only stress, also our dietary habits must pose the question of whether they influence our regenerative cells in a positive or negative manner. A balanced dietary pattern is an extremely important factor in the control of cancer and equally so in the ultimate prevention of cancer.

Although still rather young at the time of my sister's birth, I nevertheless retain some vivid memories of that period. Our general practitioner had recommended a second opinion and therefore my sister would have to be examined by a specialist at the provincial hospital.

In those dark days of the war, travel was virtually impossible as there were few means of transport remaining for civilians. As our local doctor realised that speedy action was necessary, he pointed out that the best way of travelling between the hospital and our town would probably be by hearse. This vehicle was obviously in frequent use on that stretch of road in those days. It was therefore arranged that my mother and her little daughter would be taken to and from hospital by the hearse, where my sister would receive radium treatment.

In later years my sister has come to realise that she made medical history, because she was among the earliest patients to receive this kind of treatment. It was by no means a pleasant situation, but of course my mother would do anything in her power to influence my sister's health favourably. My father had been deported by the Germans and as a result she had to tackle this problem virtually alone and she shouldered it courageously.

The treatment was effective, but we must remember that each cells grows, reproduces and then dies. Therefore a dead cell which has been removed must be replaced by a new cell, and here problems were encountered. As a result of the radium treatment many healthy cells were destroyed as well as cancerous cells and the specialist in charge of my sister's treatment made a remark, later repeated to me by my mother, which showed a great deal of vision and insight for those days. He informed my mother that in his opinion the condition of her baby was the result of a one-sided food pattern — or to put it in better English, an imbalanced food pattern. According to the specialist my sister was a product of the war when so few foodstuffs were available.

Looking back, this remark must have been revolutionary, as orthodox medicine, especially in those days, unfortunately did not pay any attention to a possible connection between food and cancer.

Unbeknown to us at that time, this eminent specialist only lived a few minutes' walk from us and I dare say that if it was not for this gentleman there might today be still more kidney problems experienced, because this specialist, Prof. Dr A. Kolf, was the inventor of the artificial kidney machine.

I was very pleased when, not long ago, I was able to watch a film shown to the staff of a hospital relating how Prof. Kolf had worked so hard during the war to establish this famous kidney machine. I only refer to this because that same eminent scientist in his time was one of the first to recognise or even consider a possible connection between cancer and food — a very revolutionary viewpoint for those days.

Although my sister was finally cured of her problem, a long list of minor illnesses plagued her right up to the age of seven, from which can be deduced that the disease and its treatment took its toll and drastically affected her immune system. Prof. Kolf had warned Mother of this possibility, but he had also told her that, with some luck, after the age of seven things could change for the better. In this statement he was also proved right. Many times I have heard my mother refer to this scientist with the greatest affection and admiration and, although in those days I was too young to appreciate it all, in my later studies I came to realise how ahead of his time he was in his theories.

During the war years the medical establishment was not ready for his insistence on a balanced food pattern. Furthermore, the means were then not available. Today, however, we realise more and more the probability of an inter-relationship between diet and cancer and leukaemia, although unfortunately the incidence of these problems is still on the increase.

It is true that during the war years, particularly during the final months, there was little food to be had in terms of *quantity*, but it is also equally true that the available food was most likely of a better *quality*. Nowadays, although the required quantity is available, often the quality is found to be lacking. Food which has been interfered with through artificial fertilisers, artificial colourings, chemical additives and preservatives, could well carry a lot of the blame for an even bigger interference with the forming of healthy cells. If the natural immune mechanism of the body is not able to remove the invaders of healthy cells, cancer cells can take over.

Under normal circumstances all cellular action occurs in an orderly way; if a cell divides in order to form a new cell and no interference takes place, nothing untoward will happen. But if outside factors are allowed to intefere a tumour may develop, which could eventually turn malignant. Then other tissues may be invaded as cells travel to other parts of the body and start new growths there. Then the forming of normal cells is endangered.

Nobody yet really knows what causes this complex disease. Modern technology and science in many fields contribute to the advance in combating certain types of cancer, but whatever is discovered often seems to increase the doubt and mystery which surrounds cancer.

All discoveries concerning the possible causes of cancer are extremely useful, but it is much more essential that lessons be learned to assist us in the *prevention* of this illness. This is especially true in today's society because of the pollution of air, food and water — the three forms of energy, vital to life.

Elimination and prevention is of the utmost importance and therefore we should concentrate on strengthening and rebuilding the immune system so that it is capable of withstanding attacks from outside interference.

As I have said, my sister's treatment was successful. She was a sickly and ailing child up to the age of seven when a considerable improvement became apparent. When the war ended Mother set to and devised a well-thought-out and sensible diet as soon as the situation allowed. She spared no effort in encouraging my sister's health to pick up and today my sister is well and healthy and she herself is the mother of two healthy sons. Occasionally when I look at her I find it hard to realise that she once suffered the after-effects of radium treatment.

In rebuilding her immune system she was given the chance to develop into a healthy person and she still follows the guidelines adhered to by our mother:

—a well-balanced and natural diet;
—no smoking or drinking.

It goes to show that it is possible for people who follow a sensible diet and who refrain from certain indulgences to control cancer or leukaemia. Moreover, I am convinced that this also goes a long way towards prevention.

I often wonder if enough investigation in this direction is being carried out. Every time I come across civilisations where cancer or leukaemia are non-existent, I must admit that they lead less stressful lives and that they generally follow sensibly balanced dietary patterns. Then I again recognise the wisdom hidden in the phrase: "We are what we eat!"

Environmental influence could be a possible factor. It is true that specific cancers seem to be more prevalent in certain parts of the world than elsewhere — for example:

—liver cancer in Africa and South East Asia;
—lung cancer in the USA and Western Europe (in the USA ascribed to catalysers in motorcars — platina!);
—stomach cancer in Japan and Chile (probably connected with too hot food);
—breast cancer in Europe and the USA (could it be due to high consumption of animal fat?);
—cancer of the womb and the mouth and throat in India and China.

Such a list leaves us wondering why these specific incidences should vary according to a seemingly geographical pattern.

It is generally believed that cancer is a disease of modern times, but in fact this is not true. In ancient Greek writings we come across references to cancer and even in the Old Testament of the Bible diseases are referred to which could well be considered as a form of cancer. Skeletons from ancient times discovered in Egypt show signs of tumours having formed. It is, however, a fact that cancer is becoming more prevalent nowadays and if we are to find a solution to this problem we must leave no stone unturned in our investigations as to the cause of this illness and better still as to its prevention.

It is doubtful if so many allergies and viruses have been encountered ever before. There remains little doubt that viruses can be a contributory factor to cancer. When viruses are diagnosed and treated properly in their early stages, much can be done for the patient. Despite all the treatments now available in both orthodox medicine as well as alternative medicine, the ones which offer the most hope are those which call upon the body's natural reserves and assist the healthy cells wherever possible to fight the abnormal cells.

I often remind patients that cancer is like warfare. It can be compared to two opposing armies: the army of degenerative cells in combat with the army of regenerative cells. If the former appears to be stronger, we have to provide the right materials and weapons for the army of regenerative cells to prop up their defences. A victory of the regenerative cells is then certainly not an impossibility.

There is a wide range of natural weapons we can use to make that army of regenerative cells stronger and in this book I will outline some of these.

Each type of cancer needs a different approach. A sarcoma — a cancer which begins in the connective tissue — will need different treatment than, for instance, a carcinoma — a cancerous growth made up of epithelial cells. A priority must be to decide on how a tumour should best be treated. It could well be the start of a neoplasm, which is an abnormal growth of tissue that can either be a benign swelling or turn out to be a malignant cancer. This malignant cancer could take the form of either a carcinoma, sarcoma or a leukaemia.

Leukaemia — cancer of the blood-forming organs and discussed in Chapter 2 — again needs a different approach. Each different form of cancer needs careful consideration and administration.

17

The basis of any approach to the different cancers mentioned has, however, to be decided on. First of all the life pattern of the patient should be scrutinised and that person should also be regarded as a complete human being, i.e. physically and mentally. Cancer actually points to the presence of a disharmony and therefore every function in the body should be taken into consideration.

It is a fact that in any case of cancer, the liver — that most efficient laboratory of the body — is always involved. The liver has some dire enemies, but thank goodness it also has a few extremely loyal friends.

Nowadays we are aware how necessary oxygen is to help the liver in the great task it performs. When the vital force in the human body is under attack, it can be aided with some of the wonderful products nature supplies to stimulate the cleansing oxygen to course through the blood. It is necessary to encourage good blood circulation in order that oxygen can be transported all through the body. How sad it is to see that so many people endanger this action by smoking and/or drinking. We only need to look at the rise in the incidence of lung cancer to realise this and one cannot get away with the statement that one's grandfather, who lived to a ripe old age, smoked most of his life. That grandfather may have been lucky, but it does not necessarily mean that his offspring is going to be equally lucky. No risks should be taken with something as vitally important as one's health.

A patient who only recently consulted me wondered why he was hit by cancer because he smoked and why it had not affected his grandfather who had lived till he was almost ninety years old and then died a peaceful death due to old age. One easily forgets that many factors play a role. I had to tell this person over and over again that his body was his own responsibility and therefore it was his duty to look after it. It is largely a question of common sense how one sets about looking for better health. To the encouragement of this gentleman, I was able to tell him that I have seen cancer which had reached even the last stage brought back to the first stage as a result of a sensible approach.

18

Despite being aware that he would not like it, I nevertheless advised him to give up smoking and drinking and follow my example and drink grape juice instead. I know that some people laugh at it, but an extremely effective remedy to restore the vital force is to eat daily a salad of freshly grated raw beetroot, carrot and apple. It is generally considered too simple to be effective, but please take this advice.

It was with great pleasure that I received a letter from a young lady in which she wrote that initially she did not like the advised diet at all and most particularly disliked beetroot. However, she had read statistics about the anti-cancerous properties of beetroot and she realised that it could mean survival to her. Needless to say she got accustomed to the taste and she was indeed rewarded because at present she enjoys much improved health.

For many years I have faithfully followed the theories of my great mentor, Alfred Vogel, and I see no reason to divert now. He is a great advocate of sensible dietary management and herbal remedies to assist the lymphatic system to cleanse the liver. I have been fortunate to witness the success of this approach and am grateful for the endless studies he has performed to this end.

He closes his latest book with the advice: "One can advise and help, but nature holds the cure. Only God the Almighty can fulfil His promise to overcome death forever."

I truly believe that if we follow the laws of nature, we obey the laws of God.

Yet, have we investigated every asset available in nature? Recently I was approached by a professor at a South African university and he pointed out that there are many plants and roots that have never yet been fully researched. One of these could well hold the answer to an effective cancer therapy. Then I am left wondering yet again why endless amounts of money have been spent on scientific research and so little effort has been made to investigate what nature may have to offer us in our battle against cancer.

Let us look at cancer from another point of view. In 1898 *The*

Lancet published an article by Dr Roger Williams in which he blamed environmental factors for the alarming increase in the death rate due to cancer in Britain. He quoted an increase from 17 to 88 people per 100,000. In comparison with today's figures we must be shocked to realise the frightful growth in these figures since then which has occurred all over the world. The present figures are obviously compiled using modern and more accurate methods and let us not show any surprise when we hear cancer sometimes referred to as "the disease of civilisation".

Cancerous growths are called tumours or neoplasms and may present themselves in many ways and in different parts of the body. When found in the cells of normal tissue, the growth is called a primary tumour. This usually occurs in tissue which in its normal function has a constant degeneration and renewal process of cells. Most primary tumours occur at locations in which there is cell renewal due to irritation or trauma.

Primary cancers, however, rarely occur in muscle or nerve tissue, where cells do not normally subdivide or renew themselves. Liver, peritoneum, lung and bone tissue are capable of supporting the growth of a secondary tumour originating from stray cells from a primary cancer elsewhere. It is unusual to perish from a primary tumour, but whenever the cancer has metastasised, the condition is often terminal.

Metastasis or a secondary cancer is formed of cells out of the primary growths, detaching and grouping together elsewhere in the body. The circulating cancer cells do not survive. For such cells to establish a secondary growth, contact with tissue is necessary in a location which is favourable and, for example, a blocked vessel, a stationary blood clot or a trauma somewhere provides a perfect place for them to settle.

When the viscosity of the blood is good and the circulation is functioning properly, the growth of the secondary cancer will be limited. Possibly now, the importance of oxygenation will be fully appreciated. The circulation of the blood can be aided by a properly balanced healthy diet and sometimes blood-thinning agents are used to obtain the right viscosity of the blood.

A specially designed diet introducing vitamins, minerals and trace elements, possibly germanium or laetrile, or some other individual remedy, may bring about a spontaneous remission from cancer. The only way in which I see recovery as a feasibility is when the immune system can be regenerated. Stimulation of the liver function and other vital organs, together with a positive attitude by the patient, can then turn the situation around.

Some important factors in the prevention of cancer are as follows:

—good oxygen supply;
—measures against constipation;
—a good blood chemistry;
—avoidance of obesity;
—exclusion of fats, high animal protein, toxic material, nicotine and alcohol from the diet;
—avoidance wherever possible of stress and pollution;
—refraining from using aluminium cooking utensils;
—making sure no deficiencies exist of vitamins, minerals and trace elements;
—avoidance of drugs (if possible);
—plenty of exercise in the fresh air;
—sparing use of salt.

Having been in practice in Scotland for the last twenty years or so, I have seen a marked increase in bowel cancer, which is considered to be about 20% higher in Scotland than elsewhere in the United Kingdom and among the highest in the world. I suppose this could possibly be due to a higher intake of alcohol, but I have also found that a surprising number of people suffer from constipation. Added to this, fat consumption is generally higher in Scotland than elsewhere.

We would do well to remember that the liver acts as a general detoxifier and therefore it deserves all possible help in its unique double-circulation system — the arterial blood supply and the portal blood circulation. The venous blood supply system returns the blood from the liver to the heart, whilst the portal system includes the veins, containing absorbed nutrients from the stomach. The duodenum and the small intestine drain into the large vessel known as the portal vein, which passes separately through the capillary blood vessels in the liver, into general circulation. The more we encourage this process — which requires common sense more than anything else — the better we can expect our health to be.

Let us not overlook the obvious: any imports must in due course be exported. It goes without saying that this ought to take place in as natural a manner as possible and without interference.

Consider the mixtures of food and drink which are often the cause of upper and lower gases, when foods ferment rather than digest: insufficient stomach acids, insufficient digestive enzymes, food soaked in alcohol so that it cannot be broken down into chemical compounds. Through these we encourage a lack of protein digestive enzymes and of hydrochloric acid, which will interfere with the normal working of all these important organs.

Cancer cannot grow when the metabolism is properly balanced. As the basic unit of life lies in the cells, let us aim to stimulate the production of healthy cells.

There are many ways in which the cellular system can be adversely affected. I am reminded of how a young person sought my advice after having been told that she had cancer. Fortunately it was discovered at an early stage. After a long talk I felt it necessary to perform an iridology test and a blood test. On checking the results of the iridology test I began to wonder about the toxicity level in her system, which indeed also showed up in the blood test. I discovered that the reason for this was dental amalgam, or silver mercury amalgam, so we decided to have all the amalgam removed from her dental fillings and replaced by composite fillings.

From the billions of cells which are continuously dividing, duplicating and dying, in order to maintain a healthy growth, it is quite possible that occasionally some of these cells become faulty. Some immunologists actually believe that we produce thousands of cancer cells, but if the immune system is healthy, there is no need to worry. Seemingly minor influences, however, such as in this case amalgam dental fillings, could play a part which should not be underestimated.

Is nature not a wonderful thing when we think that a baby originates from one cell only, created by fusion of a female ovum with male sperm! That cell multiplies to sixty trillion cells and it is reckoned that each gram of human tissue contains about one hundred million cells. Consider the responsibility of looking after these healthy cells in order to keep on top of malignant cells. Nature will gratefully accept any help offered in this task!

Not so long ago I was visited by a young man who suffered from a melanoma, a malignant neoplasm. His skin was in a dreadful condition and it is quite possible that he contracted this in the Middle East while working in the harsh sunshine. I decided on his treatment and so far the results are very encouraging. He was a sun worshipper and very proud of his tan. My advice, however, was to avoid the sun as much as possible and once I had managed to convince him, he fully co-operated. Since then his skin has improved tremendously and it is wonderful to see nature restore the damaged skin, as on the affected parts healthy skin is beginning to reappear.

This process is still continuing and thus we realise that often only minor adjustments are needed to effect recovery. In this case it required some adjustment in his diet, high dosages of additional Vitamin E plus Vitamin C, the herbal remedies Petasan and Viscasan from Alfred Vogel's range, which have as the main ingredient *Viscum album* or mistletoe. He also took some selenium and drank three glasses of raw beetroot juice daily. So often over the years I have advised cancer patients to either drink the juice of raw beetroot or to eat a beetroot salad as I described earlier.

It was a long time ago that I met a doctor in Germany who had scientifically studied the properties of beetroot. It is important that fresh raw beetroot is used and not, as is the tendency in Britain, beetroot that has been pickled or soaked in vinegar.

As part of my training in China I was instructed in facial diagnosis, which is widely practised there. I find myself subconsciously doing this quite frequently, as was the case when a new patient was shown into my consulting rooms.

It concerned a lady of about the age of forty. During our interview I studied her closely, but I was left slightly puzzled. I could not quite decide about this lady and therefore I decided to perform an iridology test. When studying the results of the test, I recognised hereditary signs of cancer in the area of the liver and the pancreas. I was not completely happy about the lungs either. When I asked about the medical history of her immediate relations, she told me that her mother had died of cancer of the liver and elsewhere in the family there had been deaths due to lung cancer and cancer of the pancreas. By no means had her condition reached an advanced stage. Particularly in such cases, iridology tests can be an extremely valuable diagnostic aid.

A slightly younger male patient had noticed some minor changes which later proved to be early signs of stomach cancer. Whereas at one stage he used to love to raid the refrigerator for anything edible, he had changed to the extent that although he still habitually opened the door of the fridge, he would only stand and look at the food without touching anything, because he had lost his appetite. He had also noticed his gums bleeding when he was cleaning his teeth.

The Dutch alternative medicine practitioner, Dr Cornelis Moerman, has listed sixteen clinical symptoms which may be very helpful in reaching a diagnosis. Let me state, however, that any of these symptoms does not automatically indicate that cancer is present, but it could serve as an early warning system if quite a few of these symptoms have been noticed. Then it is possible that a pre-cancerous state has been reached.

1. Dryness of the skin. Excessive hard skin on the soles of the feet. Hard grains in the pores of the skin. Scaly areas on the skin. Frequently a change in the colour of the skin into a sallow complexion.

2. A change in the colour of the tongue and the inside of the lips into a deeper red.

3. Chapped skin around the corners of the mouth.

4. Scaly rings around the wings of the nose.

5. Hard and brittle nails, sometimes showing stripes on the surface.

6. Dull hair where a healthy gloss has disappeared.

7. Changes in the mucous membranes noticeable with the use of a magnifying-glass.

8. A certain amount of fluid retention on the inside of the lower limbs, which could also be sensitive to touch.

9. Bleeding of the gums during the brushing of teeth.

10. A marked increase in the occurrence of bruises, even on light contact.

11. Slower healing process of wounds and forming of superfluous and inferior tissue in the wound.

12. Apathy, listlessness and a marked decrease in vitality.

13. Increase in inexplicable tiredness, experienced even before starting a task or activity.

14. Loss of appetite, which may result in loss of weight.

15. Blood defects such as anaemia, alkalinity or increased sedimentation.

16. General health and possible hereditary factors such as the occurrence of cancer in the family.

There are of course other ways of detecting cancer in its early stages, but great care is necessary in reaching the correct diagnosis and to this end blood tests are essential.

I would like to refer back to the lady whose medical family

history showed various deaths due to cancer. Fortunately in her case we managed to detect her problems at an early stage and I prescribed germanium for her and high dosages of vitamins, minerals and trace elements. I also decided on some interferon to help her quickly.

Interferon has been known to be of tremendous help in certain types of cancer and is mainly obtained from leucocytes — small, colourless cells in the blood, lymph and tissues, which are important in the body's defences against infection. Interferon obtained from white blood cells has also proved to be effective with various cancers. Sometimes a combination of two or even three types of interferon is used in the more advanced cancer stages. Immune interferon is sometimes used in the treatment of leukaemia.

At times a practitioner must have an open mind as to the treatment necessary for each particular patient. There are no hard and fast rules as to which treatment specifically combats a particular disease. Obviously there are guidelines to be followed, but the practitioner must remain flexible and at all times consider the patient as an individual and investigate the background of that person.

I remember a taxi-driver from the Midlands, whose breathing was badly affected. I was extremely worried about him and realised that the high toxicity in his system was due to lead poisoning. It was discovered that he had a cancer in a rather advanced state. To help him quickly, I used laetrile and germanium and on top of that I prescriped Ipe Roxo, from which I think he received most benefit.

Ipe Roxo is a herbal tea, made from the inner bark of the lapacho tree from southern Brazil. Another name for this remedy is Pau d'Arco. Both the tea and the paste made from the bark have been used for centuries by the Indians of Brazil for a variety of ailments, including skin cancer.

About twenty years ago it was discovered by the non-Indian community and used in the treatment of cancer when there was no other hope. Since the early sixties the Municipal Hospital of San André has experimented with the bark in the treatment of terminal cancer patients and has reported positive results. Interestingly, it was also found that the bark cured other afflictions such as diabetes. Another of the positive effects of the tea was that it appeared to relieve the pain of the sufferers.

I also prescribed for this same taxi-driver a Rumanian remedy rich in certain trace elements, called Beres drops. Certain biological processes are specific in respect of their metallic ion requirements. This means that a metallic ion in a certain state is capable of taking part in the biological reactions or is able to form the adequate stereo-structure.

The so-called essential elements are absolutely necessary for the human and animal organisms as well as for the life of plants. Those elements, which are required in small quantities only, e.g. mcg/g or less, are called trace elements. The trace elements such as copper, selenium, chromium, manganese, cobalt, etc., are suitable catalysts in enzyme reactions and have a complex relationship with hormones and vitamins. They play a role in the structural formation of bone and other tissues.

In order to compensate micro-element deficiencies or disorders due to these, Beres drops are prescribed, since they contain those micro-elements, which are important — according to our present knowledge — for the undisturbed function of the human body.

Not long after I first saw the taxi-driver, his wife wrote to let me know that the knife-like pains in his chest had started to subside within approximately twelve hours of taking the medication. The Rumanian remedy plus the herbal tea were beginning to bring relief. Later he himself let me know that his specialist was very pleased to see him looking so well and that the cancer seemed to be well contained. He added that he hoped to come back and see me in a few months' time.

I had also instructed him on breathing exercises which were necessary for him, and told him that controlled normal breathing was the highest form of regaining energy in the cells. This is of special importance for lung cancer patients.

This reminds me of another patient with lung cancer. This

time it concerned an elderly lady. She told me that she had noticed an improvement after taking ginseng. This is not surprising as ginseng contains a lot of germanium, which is also the case with garlic, barley, comfrey and bitter aloe. It is very interesting to see that such energy-giving products will also help the breathing of these patients, because of the extra oxygen produced by the germanium content of these products.

I was very pleased to hear from this elderly lady a few months later that her health was so much better. Although she had previously undergone an operation on the lymph glands, this fresh outbreak of cancer after two years was now under control. Nineteen years before she had undergone a mastectomy. It was worth while remembering how this lady had been able to control the cancer with dietary management backed up by several natural remedies.

Sadly, though, not every patient responds to treatment. I was sorry for the gentleman whom I recently saw about a very bad pain in his arm. When I examined him, I felt a familiar anxiety. I referred him to the X-ray department, but unfortunately the X-rays only confirmed my suspicions that he was in a serious condition and the secondaries in the arm were possibly as bad as the primary. Indeed, this poor man died within six weeks from cancer of the liver.

Unfortunately, as I have said before, the secondaries are mostly much more serious than the primaries, though sometimes overlooked. Such was the case with the gentleman who came to me about complaints with his knee. X-rays had already been taken, which had shown nothing out of the ordinary and certainly no secondaries had been diagnosed. When he came to me I decided on further X-rays and, unfortunately, we then realised that the situation was serious. I advised him to see his own general practitioner as soon as possible. The condition was so drastic that the leg had to be amputated. Even then it appeared that the primary cancer was so far advanced, that after a few months this gentleman unfortunately died.

Thank goodness this is not always the case. I have a letter in front of me from a lady who had an operation on secondary cancer and immediately afterwards she started therapy to strengthen her immune system. After a period of six weeks she wrote to me to say how much better she felt and asked for a repeat prescription of the blood-thinning medication and Echinaforce, a natural antibiotic from Vogel. She also took a high dosage of Vitamin C and some Petasan, another Vogel preparation. These were the only remedies she used, alongside a well-balanced healthy diet.

There was also the young baby twin. Her parents had looked into every possibility to find a way of dealing with an inoperable brain tumour. They were totally nonplussed as to why this should become apparent in such a young child and why in one of the twins, while the other was healthy.

Unfortunately we are not able to give an answer to that question, as it is a mystery to all of us. One thing we do know, however, is that more children are struck by cancer than ever before. According to an article in the *Observer* of Sunday 1 December 1985, higher rates of leukaemia and cancer in children have been discovered near nuclear power stations. In the area surrounding the Holy Loch nuclear submarine base, the incidence of cancer is triple that of the average Scottish cancer rate among under-25s. Over the past fifteen years leukaemia has increased fivefold in the area of Windscale.

Both cancer and leukaemia are more prevalent than ever before to our knowledge. We are still very much in the dark as to the reasons for this, but possibly some have already been dealt with in this chapter.

The pattern of a cancer's development is variable and it can take a long time before cancer comes to a crisis point. Some cancers can develop very slowly and lie dormant for twenty or thirty years, while others will develop very quickly and spread like mushrooms. The former was the case with my father.

My father had always been a healthy man and had never had anything wrong with him. He was both a mentally and physically well-balanced person until the war came. I will

29

never forget seeing him on his return from the Nazi labour camp. His weight was so low that it seemed as if some skin had been carelessly draped over his bones. But we were delighted that he had survived and my mother did everything within her power to help him regain his health.

I remember the day so well when, nearly thirty years later, he came and told me that he had not been feeling well for some time. He was not able to eat because he would immediately feel sick and he wondered what could be wrong. I told him that he should see the doctor and I would accompany him. Our general practitioner also happened to be our next-door neighbour and my father explained the situation to him.

Sadly the doctor's reactions confirmed my suspicions. I went with my father to the hospital for further examination. Unfortunately, in those days I did not know about the many alternative treatments with which I work nowadays. My father agreed to undergo the operation which was deemed necessary as he could only accept food if it was administered intravenously.

Although the primary cancer was found to be in the stomach, secondaries had metastasised right up into the chest. The cancer had grown like a climber and spread wildly. The surgeon did his utmost in removing the secondaries, but could not give us any guarantee as to how successful he had been in locating all the secondaries and whether it would stir up again.

The surgeon was totally open about the situation and answered all my questions truthfully. When I enquired how long this condition might have been in existence, he answered that it could possibly have been building up to this over the last twenty or thirty years. The stressful time my father had experienced under the Nazi regime had possibly claimed another victim.

If my father had not followed such a healthy lifestyle since the war years, the cancer would not have remained dormant for so long. We had reason to be grateful that he had survived on borrowed time for so many years and I am convinced that this was largely due to my mother's sensible administrations.

After that operation my father lived only for another six months. He made the best of it and there is no doubt that it was because of his recovered immune system that he lasted so long.

The lesson of this, however, is that the cancer cells could very likely have been controlled even longer, if we had known then about some of the methods we use today in alternative medicine. Isn't it sad to think that for all the money spent on scientific cancer research, we discover more and more alternative ways of approaching the cancer problem!

Hence the title of this book: *Cancer and Leukaemia — An Alternative View*.

In this book I have set out to describe some of the different methods used throughout the world for the prevention and treatment of cancer.

2

What is Leukaemia?

LEUKAEMIA is a disease of the blood-forming organs resulting in an abnormal increase in the production of leucocytes. The reason I single out leukaemia from the many cancers we know has already been touched upon in the previous chapter, namely the alarming increase in this disease among the younger generation. Especially because it seems to affect young people, it causes a great deal of worry and pain, and this has urged me to make further studies in this particular condition in an effort to find ways in which we possibly can protect the younger generation.

By now we must be aware of how much our reserves and our immune system — in other words our general health — are under threat in our present society. Outside influences can so easily disturb our innate energy and imbalance positive and negative reactions.

Leukaemia, as a cancer of the blood-forming organs and the bone-marrow, is characterised by the abnormal increase of white corpuscles in the blood. It causes the blood-producing organs to let loose large numbers of primitive lymphocytes in the blood, otherwise called polymorphonuclear leucocytes. There also exist leukaemias caused by increased numbers of monocytes or eosinophils in the circulatory system. Even though there are diverse names for the various forms of this disease, I will continue to use the collective term of leukaemia.

No one can be certain about the cause of leukaemia, but over the years I have come to believe that mental influences very likely play some role here as well.

I remember a great friend of the family who was not only enormously popular with my brother and sister and myself, but equally appreciated by my parents. He had a great influence in our development, because of his personality, and I retain fond memories of him. We used to have long talks and I imagine that he can be credited as one of my most influential teachers spiritually.

Unfortunately, we lost him while he was still only middle-aged and yet my memories of him are always of a strong and healthy person. No one ever asked him for help and came away disappointed, he was always ready for anyone who sought advice or help.

He had not been feeling too well for a while and went to see his doctor, who referred him to the hospital for tests. I will never forget that he had been given a letter for the specialist and on his way to that appointment he called in for a cup of coffee. I can still remember him sitting there at the table and fingering the envelope containing the letter for the specialist and voicing his fears that he instinctively realised that he was handling his death certificate. How right he turned out to be!

He returned after his interview with the specialist who had told him — and now I speak of quite some years back — that very little could be done for leukaemia.

His specialist was in those days a highly regarded scientist who grew to be famous in his chosen field of medicine. This gentleman took our dear friend through his medical history, from which no indicative cause could be pinpointed. They talked at length and then he hit on the possibility of a great emotional trauma.

During the war he had visited friends on a nearby island and while returning home their boat had come under severe attack from the Germans. It had seemed a miracle at the time that the lives of himself and one of his friends had been saved. He had, however, been so shocked by the death and destruction around him that for a number of days he had acted out of character. When the specialist heard about this, he was quite sure that such a traumatic experience could cause a drastic disturbance in his natural energies, that it could possibly have been a trigger point for a physical reaction, i.e. in his case perhaps leukaemia.

The details of his suffering and death are not relevant here, but nowadays I often wish that I had known then about germanium, because it would have eased the drawn-out process so much for him.

However, when I was asked much later to take on the treatment of a young girl, I had fortunately become aware of the fine properties of germanium, which I will discuss in detail in Chapter 5. Although her condition was terminal, it was possible to use this to comfort her in her suffering.

There are so many questions to be asked in relation to leukaemia. In his book *The Health Revolution*, my good friend Ross Horne writes that back in 1961 the Communicable Diseases Center of the United States Public Health Service in Atlanta reported that a certain school in Niles, Illinois, had the highest rate of leukaemia of any school in the country. In fact, it was five times the national average.

I have had the pleasure of listening to several lectures given by Dr John Ott, from Florida, USA. He has studied the possibility of any relation between colours, infra-red rays, fluorescent light and other radiation influences and the occurrence of cancer and leukaemia.

Dr Ott personally visited the Illinois school and interviewed the teaching staff. From them he learned that the children who had developed leukaemia were located in two classrooms. Because the windows in these particular classrooms were shielded by greenish translucent curtains, warm white fluorescent light had been provided, which had a strong, orange-pink spectrum. He wondered if this could be considered as a common factor in the incidences of leukaemia. On his advice the decoration was changed and the situation began to improve.

He had reached this conclusion by looking for similarities in the children and their surroundings, both at home as well as at school. Although it was known that the endocrine system is sensitive to sunlight and artificial rays, no association with cancer had previously been reported.

The pineal gland, which is sometimes referred to as the "third eye", thrives on ultra-violet rays. However, it is not very fond of infra-red or artificial rays, which can cause damage. In cases of leukaemia, the endocrine system deserves extra consideration, but unfortunately not enough in-depth study into these small glands has yet taken place.

What we do know is that these glands can be influenced positively and they prefer surroundings to be as natural as possible. For instance, the role of natural light associated with leukaemia in schoolchildren and the influence on the pineal and endocrine glands are now receiving serious study.

The X-ray technique was a great invention for medical science and it is of tremendous value in reaching or confirming a diagnosis, but we also know that X-rays could be a causative factor in cancer. Nowadays, with the help of modern technology, X-ray equipment has been redesigned in order to cut this risk to the minimum and also more preventive measures are taken. X-rays are capable of destroying white blood cells in the bloodstream and these are extremely important for protection against foreign intruders. Although they are sometimes unavoidable, I always advise my own patients to keep X-rays to the very minimum.

The radiotherapist Carl Simonton realised that this risk existed when listening to a lecture by the prominent immunologist who had experimented with leukaemic patients. In this lecture he related some of the remarkable results he had obtained with vaccinations to stimulate the immune system.

Simonton heard about the resulting regression and was so excited by this immunologist's discovery that he pondered as to what extent positive thinking could be applied here.

Personally I feel that Simonton's mind control and visualisation techniques are of great value for the endocrine system, if practised correctly. The endocrine system appears to be so sensitive to emotion, vision and vibration, that with these techniques clear and positive reactions can be obtained. In the last chapter of this book I intend to discuss some of these practical mind-over-matter techniques in some detail.

As I have already mentioned in relation to cancer generally, it is also advisable for leukaemia patients to follow a well-balanced healthy diet and to introduce extra vitamins, minerals and trace elements. It was interesting to see that during an eight-month trial of a magnesium-deficient diet, a laboratory rat developed leukaemia. Similar tests produced corresponding results due to a shortage of selenium in the diet.

I feel that such research justifies my insistence on a properly balanced diet. Added to this I must stress that we should never let the prevention factor out of sight. The old adage "prevention is better than cure" contains a lot of wisdom.

An article published in The Lancet, written by T. Allan Philips, states that in 1957 leukaemia in Britain was five times higher than it was in 1920. After the well-known Windscale nuclear reactor accident the incidence of leukaemia rose over the next five years to thirty-six times the previous national average. The question now is what this figure will be in a few years' time as a result of the fallout following the Chernobyl disaster.

I have explained the relationship between leukaemia and the endocrine system. Lymphatic leukaemia arises from primary malignancy of the lymphatic system. In these cases the circulating blood contains an immense number of lymphocytes. High dosages of Vitamin C, calcium and kelp can be of great help here. It is known that the symptoms of an acute leukaemia are almost identical to those of scurvy and therefore Vitamin C is essential for a healthy lymphocyte production.

When chemotherapy has been suggested, it is advisable to assist the cellular system with extra vitamins, minerals and trace elements to aid the production of new cells.

Basically, leukaemia is different from the many cancers we know, because we are up against a progressive process in the white blood cells.

The old and established principle of "pure foods, pure water and pure air" certainly gives us food for thought.

3

Cancer and the Immune System

SOME TIME AGO, during a lecture in Canada, my co-lecturer was Linus Pauling — twice Nobel Prize winner — who stressed the importance of the immune system and its relation to the use of Vitamin C.

I was very happy with that lecture as it underlined so many of my own thoughts gathered over the years. I could not help thinking back to how the Canadians liberated us in the Netherlands at the end of World War II. We were so happy to see them arrive in our part of the country after the misery and suffering of the "Hungerwinter". Then everything seemed so bleak with little hope for the future.

At the age of eight I weighed approximately two and a half stones and my health was in dire straits. How grateful we were for the help we got from the Red Cross, who distributed seemingly insignificant little tablets containing Vitamin C. I am quite sure that those little tablets were rightly regarded as a godsend and life-savers. These enabled us to keep our immune systems ticking over till the end of the war, keeping us alive to enjoy the liberation by the Allied Forces.

When I see the present generation of Canadians spoiling themselves with all the wrong foods, and consider their enormous consumption of chocolate, I wish they would think back and realise once again the value of Vitamin C in particular. I wish, too, that they would pay more attention to a natural and healthy diet in general — and that really is the message I deliver in any lecture I give anywhere in the world.

It seems to me that never before in history have we needed to focus more on the immune system than at present. With cancer and leukaemia it is clear that the more we strengthen the immune system and our own natural reserves, the more chance of survival we have. I have been surprised many times in clinics which I have visited all over the world, that when attention is directed to a good diet, the survival rate rises.

Today, not only with cancer and leukaemia, but with any disease and especially infectious diseases, it is of great importance that we nurture and care for our immune system. But what really is the immune system?

The body's immune system includes three main types of immune cell:

—B-lymphocytes;
—T-lymphocytes;
—macrophages (scavenger cells).

All B-lymphocyte cells are made from bone-marrow and are responsible for the production of antibodies. However, all three types of immune cells found in the body work together in attacking bacteria, foreign invaders and toxic substances, such as cancer and viruses.

In order for the immune system to develop properly and be able to combat cancer cells, not only natural proteins are needed, but also the essential amino-acids — for adults and children alike. Also necessary are Vitamins A, B_5, B_6, B_{12} and C, iron, folic acid, biotin, selenium, zinc, pantothenic acid, magnesium, copper and essential fatty acids such as GLA (gammoleic acid) or oil of evening primrose (EPA). All these substances are capable of boosting the immune system.

39

Vitamin A helps to regulate the system and a lack of it will cause a deficiency in T-lymphocyte cells. The B vitamins will help to increase the production of thymus hormone.

Linoleic acid is needed to support the essential fatty acids. Evening primrose oil, together with linoleic acid, will help the levels of the prostaglandin, which also helps the T-lymphocyte cells in the immune system.

In the thymus glands of young animals substances are formed that have the ability to transform lymphocytes. So-called T-lymphocytes recognise the bacteria and viruses that have invaded the cells and attack them. Alien albumen and degenerated cells are likewise rendered innocuous through this defence mechanism.

In the human organism after puberty the thymus gland gradually reduces the level of production of these substances which are so important for defence. By the age of forty the activity of the gland will have fallen to about 10% of its original level. As evidence of this inadequacy, immunity and auto-immunity diseases, such as rheumatism and cancer, appear with increasing frequency. The regular replacement of thymus hormones can therefore counteract the genesis of diseases of old age and enable the already diseased organism to react in defence. It is also known that zinc deficiency minimises the lymphocyte function in the immune system.

Other influences can deplete the immune system and cause a breakdown within the cells. Where there is a lack of the required amino acids the malignant tissue will further degenerate because of insufficient support resulting from an incomplete protein chain of amino acids.

In our battles to overcome cancer we hear more and more about possible stimulation of the immune system, which is a powerful as well as complex defence mechanism for the body to ward itself against foreign matter and invading viruses, bacteria and parasites. If kept in good order the immune system is equally capable of absorbing and destroying cancer cells.

When I have needed to stimulate the complex action of the

40

immune system, I have found interferon, germanium and laetrile to be invaluable.

Immunity is the degree of resistance that a body can muster to a type of invading micro-organism resulting from:

—inheritance;
—having an attack of that particular infection;
—vaccination or some other artificial means of preventing a disease.

Immunity is due to the presence of antibodies. Antibodies are proteins present in the blood and antigens are substances that stimulate the production of antibodies or react with them.

Antibodies can originate naturally or spontaneously or be acquired through vaccination etc. Harmful micro-organisms, invading the body, act as antigens and stimulate the production of antibodies, which oppose their activities. Antibodies are specific in their reaction, directing it only against a particular kind of micro-organism or even a particular strain of it. When an organism invades the body, appropriate antibodies may already exist, and if they are present in adequate amounts the infected person will not develop the disease.

If a micro-organism does invade the body, antibodies to it are produced in about ten days. Once this has taken place, these are likely to remain indefinitely in the blood and may thus prevent a person suffering a second attack of that particular infection.

It is therefore unusual for a person to have a second attack of mumps, for example, because there is a considerable antibody reaction to this infection; conversely, it is very usual for a person to have many attacks of the common cold, to which the antibody reaction is minimal.

A child acquires some antibodies from its mother if she has had a particular infection, as these can be transmitted to the child *in utero*. These antibodies can usually prevent a newly born child from getting that particular infection, but they mostly disappear within a few weeks, leaving the child open to attack.

41

The action of the immune system can be approximately divided into three separate actions or happenings.

Initially there is an enlargement of the adrenal cortex. The hormones produced by this part of the adrenal gland assist the normal body functions in times of stress. In order to produce more hormones to cope with the increased demand, the gland increases in size. If the stress of over-production continues for too long, the gland cannot keep pace and eventually loses its ability to produce enough hormones.

Then there is a shrinkage in the lymphatic tissue, which, as we know, is actively involved with the production of immune cells. Then a specific type of immune cell may disappear completely from the body.

Finally, there may also be ulcerations in the lining of the stomach and the duodenum. These may in themselves be only minor, but nevertheless potentially dangerous and even life-threatening.

When foreign matter or antigens manage to invade the body, the immune system responds in a specific way. The humoral response system synthesises and secretes antibodies compatible to the intruding antigen, whilst the cell-mediated immune system responds by making and releasing cells in the particular antigen. The humoral response system acts against bacterial infection and viral re-infections.

The B-lymphocytes play a major role in the immune system and it is not that long ago since scientists first managed to separately identify two kinds of lymphocytes, i.e. T-cells and B-cells. Each acts separately. It is known that the T-cells and the B-cells both originate in the bone-marrow and nowadays it is also known that the lymphocytes migrate to reach that mature stage.

The macrophages or scavenger cells attach themselves to tissue and are transported by the blood. They are on their guard for harmful substances. It is well known that cancer cells will suppress a normal immune response. Tumours often grow in the presence of a defective immune system. Although it is a complex process, it is also true that interactions of direct cell contact with oxygen, nutrients, ions and other agents, can influence this process.

It is, however, equally possible for cancer cells to escape the immune system and establish themselves elsewhere. This means that cancer cells which have escaped destruction, have escaped detection by the immune system.

It is important for the immune system that regular detoxification takes place and thereto good bowel movement is essential. It is sometimes claimed that many cancers originate from the bowels and I always inform relevant patients accordingly. My great-grandmother's advice was that, if necessary, one should use castor-oil to avoid any danger of constipation. Fortunately, more palatable means to this end are nowadays available to us.

Often the question arises of how the immune complex damage occurs and here several factors could be relevant. More important to the practitioner, however, is that immune complexes of the appropriate type must be indicated in the tissue or the organ. An accurate assessment of the damage due to immune complex disease is important in order to decide which disease has attacked the immune system.

A disease could well result from a minor infection, inhalation of antigenic dust, or ingestion of any unsuitable matter in food and drink. The monitoring of the immune system is of great importance and fortunately today we have various types of apparatus and devices which prove helpful in this.

The possibilities of identifying the cause of any attack on the immune system offers great scope for the future and for further research. Since 1950 trials have been continuously undertaken to assess how vaccination and immunisation can influence the immune system.

Among its many functions, the thymus gland also forms the hormone peptide. Throughout life T-lymphocytes are engaged in permanent defensive action, constantly influenced by health and illness.

The thymus gland is located under the breastbone and from

there it directs the lymphocytes to where they are needed and deploys them as key operatives to the immune system. Production of lymphocyte cells occurs in the bone-marrow, thymus, spleen, tonsils, adenoids and in the lymphoid tissue found in the small intestine.

The soft tissue in the hollows of the long bones of arms and legs, known as the bone-marrow, produces cells which are destined to migrate as they continue to multiply. They progress to become the immuno-commutant, or to produce immunity. Through this intricate computerised mechanism the lymph nodes also bring together the specialised co-operating functions needed to produce immunity.

Lymph nodes are small, compact structures lying in groups along the course of the lymphatic vessels, and its network is comparable to the system of blood vessels. It should therefore be understood that the lymphatic system plays an important preventative and defensive role.

I have already remarked on the fact that the thymus gland slowly shrinks into disappearance. You may be interested to see the appropriate figures that back up this process:

—a newly born baby has about 1 to 1.5 million cells in the thymus;
—at the age of twenty this will be reduced to 700,000 cells;
—this figure will have decreased to about 250,000 in a forty-year-old

Considering the importance of these cells to our immune system one must agree that any stimulation of these cells is fully justified. Nothing can be done to reverse the shrinking process of the thymus gland, but extra care of all the endocrine glands, specifically the thyroid gland, will not go amiss.

It is no exaggeration to refer to the thymus gland as the "braincentre" for the whole of the immune system. If this is weak, it will easily fall prey to viruses and allergies. It has also become generally accepted that if there is a weakening of hormonal reactions, the immune system also suffers. This more or less translates into the requirement that all endocrine glands be in harmony with each other. It was shown in recent research that not only the thyroid but also the pituitary gland related closely to the activation of the immunoglobulin.

One of my favourite sayings often used in lectures is "Illness is disharmony". Anything in the human system that goes out of harmony will cause problems. Could it be a coincidence that the solar spectrum consists of seven basic colours and that there are seven endocrine glands? Never mind how small and insignificant these glands may seem, minor changes can cause either positive or negative deviations.

It has already been mentioned that cancer need not necessarily be caused by physical reasons, but can also be induced by a mental attitude. Emotions, stress and trauma greatly influence the endocrine glands. This explains the increasing popularity of holistic medicine. Unfortunately this approach is still regarded as unorthodox, yet here the patient is treated as a whole and complete being and every aspect of him and his life is studied to obtain a complete picture of him.

Certain forms of meditation such as prayer and visualisation techniques are practised with the view to the endocrine system, which then create a good hormonal balance.

Science still has no full understanding of the hormonal workings of the endocrine system. It is time that in-depth research was undertaken relating to this but I wonder if any allowance in previous research has been made in relation to the mental aspect.

Let us have another look at the pineal gland. There is little doubt that this gland or "third eye", as it is sometimes called, is definitely influenced by stress, prayer and meditation. At the same time it is true that we don't yet know enough about the medical or physical aspect of the pineal gland. This gland, by means of acupuncture, can be balanced positively or negatively. In stressful situations, when working on this particular gland, the results can be very rewarding.

The pituitary gland is said to be the key to the chemistry of the whole of the body. The pituitary hormones chemically affect the cell membranes. Therefore the chemical reactions do not work properly when the pituitary gland is in any way impaired or prevented from doing its correct job. Good protein intake, in other words good vegetable protein, is most important for the production of hormones, and also the different enzymes in the body. If the enzyme production is insufficient, the hormone balance will fail the immune system.

The pituitary gland is often also referred to as the master gland or conductor of the endocrine orchestra, and it releases hormones to either promote or inhibit the release of other endocrine hormones. Indirectly it controls such basic processes as rate of growth, metabolic rate, water and electrolyte balance, kidney filtration, ovulation and lactation. It responds to hormones released by the region of the brain known as the hypothalamus, and is a physical link between the nervous and the endocrine system.

The thyroid is a glandular link between the brain and the reproductive organs and it is certain that the thyroid can be triggered or inhibited by emotional disturbances, directly influencing circulation, respiration, tissue growth and repair. Over production of thyróxine from the thyroid gland will lead to problems and, equally, so will under-production. We often see how individuals are emotionally affected when a defect appears.

The pancreas secretes digestive enzymes into the small intestine, which produces hormones for release into the blood. The digestive enzymes are crucial because the incorrect breakdown of ingested fats, proteins and sugars can lead to digestive complaints, e.g. diabetes or hypoglycaemia. The islets of Langerhans — a group of cells within the pancreas — secrete insulin into the blood and so influence the level of glucose in the body. The pancreas also plays an important role in regulating the hormonal balance.

When we realise that the adrenals produce fifty different natural steroid hormones, we recognise the importance of these glands. Some of these hormones are involved in the conversion of dietary protein and fat into glucose, while others suppress inflammation and promote healing. Yet another group regulates the blood/iron balance in the kidneys and still others affect the sex functions. The principal hormone produced, called adrenaline, will be ready to respond to any emergencies.

The gonads — male and female sexual endocrine glands — are for the reproduction of the species. At puberty the hormones aid development of the secondary sexual characteristics of the male and female bodies and activate their reproductive systems. Another role lies in securing harmony between all the endocrine glands. We see too often in cases of stress or menopausal problems how these glands will play an enormous role, physically as well as mentally.

It is well known that poor nutrition will affect the sexual glands and that the functions of the vital organs will be impaired if the diet is lacking proper nutrition. All in all, it becomes clear that these apparently insignificant and small glands have an enormous effect on the well-being of the immune system. Overall health care is therefore extremely important.

I have already touched upon whether it could be a coincidence that there are seven endocrine glands as there are seven basic colours in the solar spectrum. It is, however, a fact that the eye possesses seven layers of light receptors. Through these the cosmic force of the seven basic colours influences the endocrine glands.

Because of the depressive aspect of the illness, a cancer patient can therefore try to turn this cosmic force in the rainbow of light and colour to their advantage, keeping a clear vision and focusing on getting better. The seven layers of light receptors in the retina of the eye serve as an indicator when practising iridology, allowing the practitioner to quickly detect disturbances. How sensitive these receptors are is clearly noticeable from observing cancer patients who over indulge in watching television, as disharmony can be caused by this.

Generally, the awareness is growing of the adverse effects of computer screens, word processors and television screens, etc. Often co-ordination problems result from over exposure to these and further study on this aspect is recommendable. By no means do I mean to imply that these screens are the cause of cancer. What I am saying is that one should remain cautious, as disharmony *can* be caused.

Each case of immune deficiency should be judged individually. The immune system can be influenced in so many ways — and several of these will be discussed in later chapters.

4

Vitamins, Minerals and Trace Elements

QUITE A FEW years ago I received a totally unexpected and unusual letter, written by an inmate from an American prison. The writer was serving a life sentence. At the time I wondered, and I still do occasionally, about what motivated this prisoner to write to me. On reading the letter I deliberated as to how I could help this person and also on what the reason was behind his desire for life. After all, when one is serving a life sentence, there seems little or no prospect for the future and therefore I was surprised by the determination of this man.

He wrote that he was the son of a Scottish dentist and as he was stricken with cancer, he had taken the liberty to write to me for advice. He had heard and read about dietary management and the use of vitamins, minerals and trace elements in the battle against cancer and it was to this end he asked for advice.

I wrote back to him with some dietary guidelines, bearing in mind that these could be difficult to introduce into the regime of prison life, but he had stated that the prison staff would not be unwilling to help. I informed him about the foods to be avoided and also listed foods that needed to be introduced into his diet.

Although I realised that it could be difficult for him to obtain certain remedies or medications, I nevertheless explained that I felt he should try and take at least 4-5g of Vitamin C daily and if possible take apricot kernels. In those days these were easily available in the USA. Otherwise, I recommended that he try to use Vitamin B_{17}, also known as laetrile.

Not long after replying to his letter I received his reply, in which he informed me that he had studied my advice and had decided to start following the recommended regime.

From the subsequent letters that were exchanged between us, it became clear that his condition showed a gradual improvement, which also became obvious to others.

When I took part in an international conference on cancer in Los Angeles, I learned that one of the lecturers there had actually visited him. He had kept notes of the prisoner's progress and insisted that these had been of great help in trials which he had conducted. These experiments and tests had been instrumental in defining possible cancer therapies.

I was delighted with his findings because laetrile, or Vitamin B_{17}, has often received unfair criticism. Pressure has been brought to bear against its use, especially by people who don't fully comprehend the role vitamins play in our daily lives. Unfortunately, the whole subject has often been treated out of context. Clinical trials have shown remarkable results and testimonials from people who have used laetrile, whether in the shape of tablets, injections or apricot kernels, make interesting reading and give us reason for sincere enthusiasm.

I have been overwhelmed by the number of people who have been prepared to testify personally during cancer conferences. They have shown willingness to talk about the changes which have taken place in their condition since using laetrile and other vitamins, minerals and trace elements in combination with a wholesome diet.

Many practitioners throughout the world have come to appreciate laetrile for what it is worth and are willing to testify as to its results. Unfortunately, other voices are equally adamant in their opposition to this remedy and therefore there is still a long way to go before the tremendous value of Vitamin B_{17} will be fully realised.

In this chapter I intend to quote some testimonials from people who have been under my care and who, thanks to careful monitoring, are still with us today. Some of these people have been under treatment for ten years or longer and they still successfully follow the programme.

One of my oldest patients must surely be the 98-year-old lady who has used laetrile for the past sixteen years in a carefully balanced dosage. In this way her condition has been kept remarkably controlled and, to the surprise of some critics, it is clear that she has not been poisoned yet! Careful handling, administration and monitoring are nevertheless essential.

Of course guidance or knowledge is necessary for everyone who uses extra vitamins, minerals and trace elements and a careful balance needs to be adhered to. This is especially the case with Vitamin C. Although it is usually said that Vitamin C has no side-effects whatsoever, to which I mostly agree, I still consider it important that when higher doses are used, this is only done under guidance of a knowledgeable doctor or nutritionist. Vitmain C is one of the most important vitamins, especially in prevention and treatment of cancer.

In the first chapter I mentioned that from personal experience I have come to appreciate the value of Vitamin C. With patients undergoing any form of treatment where Vitamin C is used, I see the beneficial results.

We have good reason to be grateful to the Nobel Prize winner Linus Pauling, who, together with the Scot Dr Ewan Cameron, has written a book on cancer and the value of Vitamin C in its treatment. Statistics show that in America every minute-and-a-half one person dies as a result of cancer. Equally elsewhere, we see the death rate from cancer and leukaemia rising at a frightful speed.

Cancer is caused by agents or conditions which bring a change in the genetic material of the cells. Many influences

51

can be considered here, but much evidence is available today that Vitamin C has a strengthening and preventive effect.

There are many types of cancer and an accurate diagnosis is absolutely essential in order that a practitioner can design a programme for the patient that is well thought out from every angle. The practitioner has to be realistic in the diagnosis of cancer and consider his goal in trying to save the life of his patient with whatever knowledge he has.

Indeed there are remedies and methods today which can ease the suffering of a cancer patient and if there is no outlook for the future for the patient, much can be done to minimise that suffering. When patients are struck by some of the more aggressive types of cancer, their suffering can be eased considerably and practitioners are obliged to bear this in mind.

Let us please understand that Vitamin C does not bring about a miraculous cure, but tests have shown how much help this simple treatment can be.

The other day a father came to see me with his three-year-old child, who had a brain tumour, and I learned that the child was receiving treatment from a well-known practitioner. On his recommendation she was taking between 10 and 15 grams of Vitamin C daily and there were no side-effects apparent.

However, the child did not receive the full benefit of this large dosage of Vitamin C, because without certain additional measures the body cannot absorb these quantities and the vitamin will leave the body within a few hours of ingestion.

Unfortunately, we seem to be living in a period when allergies and viruses are rife. I meet people who have become so obsessed with allergies that they visit one allergy specialist after another. In this process they not only spend an unnecessary amount of money, but they also tend to become confused by the various recommendations given as a result of allergy tests.

When a mother came to me recently with her young child, consider my astonishment when I was forced to reach a diagnosis which was practically unthinkable in the present

52

day and age. As a result of the conflicting information received she had refrained from giving her child so many different foods that I found the child suffering from scurvy, the dreaded disease of olden days, which is due to a deficiency of Vitamin C.

Vitamin C is present in so many good nutritious foods, but where these foods are excluded problems can easily occur. Such was the case here and this poor girl had become the victim of self-doctoring without the supervision and guidance of a specialist. Such problems are of course totally unnecessary nowadays.

While preparing this chapter I received a letter from a patient who lives quite far from here which cheered me up tremendously. She wrote:

"Dear Dr de Vries, Two years ago I wrote to you enquiring about an alternative medical approach and I received a very encouraging and informative reply.

"I can inform you now that I have followed your advice and have managed to stay well since, while leading a busy and fulfilling life. It is almost three years now since I had breast cancer and I feel fit and well. I take the recommended vitamins regularly and I also think that attitude is one of the greatest things in containing this condition.

"I take great pleasure in being able to send you, in the healthiest of ways, my sincere greetings."

There now seems to be a plethora of food unlike ever before. In my opinion, however, we remain basically too careless about what we eat. Then of course, there is the problem of declining soil quality, resulting in nutrition being drained from the food. On top of that it seems to be fashionable to refine our food unnecessarily, add preservatives and chemical colourings in many cases — and all this will result in poorer nutritional value. Therefore the role of vitamins is possibly more important now than previously.

The way we have tampered with our food and have rendered it deficient in nutritional value is detrimental in our battle against cancer and leukaemia.

Dr Raymond J. Schamberger PhD, who is based at the famous Cleveland Clinic, a top research facility in the USA, is of the opinion that the risk of cancer can be reduced by 50% if one eats wholesome foods and takes vitamins A, C and E and the mineral selenium. Many practitioners are convinced that these vitamins are useful in the prevention of cancer.

One of the most important factors is that Vitamin C destroys nitrate, a cancer-causing agent in food. By taking Vitamin C in several smaller dosages spread over the day, a better effect can be expected due to the absorption problems already mentioned.

The general rule is that vitamins should be taken at meal times. Vitamins A, C and E together with selenium are indeed powerful weapons against cancer and it has been proven that Vitamin E and selenium together prevent tumours in animals.

Vitamin E is beneficial in most causes of skin tumours and also breast cancer. All this, of course, is to be done in conjunction with good dietary management and close supervision of vitamin intake.

Several times I have had the pleasure of meeting Dr William Donald Kelley, who has done a lot of work on metabolic awareness. After long years of study, he has designed a programme called "Metabolic Typing — Medicine's Missing Link". This is a system devised for identifying the inherited biochemical and neurological patterns of strengths and weaknesses that are unique to each individual, and how these strengths and weaknesses respond to lifestyle and environmental influences

The function of maintaining life is called metabolism — the total exchange of energy with the environment, an exchange involving food, water, air, light, heat, etc. How a person uses these raw materials to maintain life differs from one person to another. These differences Dr Kelley refers to as the concept of Metabolic Nutritional Individuality. This concept has been expanded on by Dr Kelley, who eventually classified the differences into ten different types of metabolism. Research has indicated that all people fall into one of these ten metabolic types, according to their Metabolic Nutritional Individuality.

According to Dr Kelley, the master regulator of the metabolism is the autonomic nervous system, which controls involuntary metabolic actions such as heartbeat and digestion. In his research over the past twenty-five years he has found that most people are neurologically influenced more strongly by either the "accelerator" (sympathetic) or "decelerator" (parasympathetic) branch of the autonomic nervous system. Everyone, he found, is different in the degree in which their bodies are influenced by these branches.

This apparently inherited tendency for varying degrees of nerve stimulation means that each individual's glands and organs, their bodies as a whole, function differently. We are as unique on a metabolic biochemical level as we are in our fingerprints. The variances in glandular and organ function result in different chemical and hormonal outputs, which in turn affects personality, physical characteristics and behaviour patterns.

Dr Kelley works according to the principle that when people have been classified into their own metabolic types, it becomes possible to determine what vitamins, minerals, foods and other supplements would best support their body chemistry. He is then able to quickly tell which supplements and foods they should not have.

In turn, the proper nutrients for the individual can be utilised by the body for the building up of all the organs and systems so that serious degenerative conditions may be prevented, or the body's own immune mechanisms be assisted to defeat them.

This theory is based on the assumption that if you give the body all the essential nutrients — everything it needs — relieve the structural problems, stimulate the glands to function efficiently, cleanse the toxins from the body regularly, and maintain a favourable mental and emotional state, the total metabolism will become more efficient. If all the organs and glands are functioning at anywhere near 100%

efficiency, the body chemistry can be rebalanced and the body will be more prepared to deal with adverse health conditions.

In one of his lectures I heard Dr Kelley state the four principles which are necessary to achieve the above:

1. Learn to apply remarkable concepts about individual nutritional, structural and emotional needs.
2. Learn to apply simple, efficient detoxifying measures that can eliminate months of accumulated toxins.
3. Learn to apply the diet and supplement programme that matches your personal metabolism.
4. Learn to apply to your own life the reality of the psychological differences between individuals and to appreciate these differences.

With few exceptions, the body is not able to synthesise vitamins, which must therefore be supplied in the diet or through dietary supplements. Vitamins are important to the body as constituents of enzymes, which function as catalysts in nearly all metabolic reactions. As such, vitamins help to regulate metabolism, convert fat and carbohydrates into energy, and assist in forming bone and tissue. Vitamins are not components of major body structures, but aid in the building of these structures. Their various functions are detailed below.

Vitamin A

Vitamin A, or carotene, is known to reduce the incidence of cancer. It can help to neutralise the action whereby a cancer cell produces a protein which inhibits the action of the immune system. One of the richest sources of Vitamin A is fish-liver oil, which is classified as a food supplement. Vitamin A aids in the growth and repair of body tissues and helps to maintain a smooth, soft skin. Internally, it helps to protect the mucous membranes of the mouth, nose, throat and lungs, thereby reducing susceptibility to infection.

Vitamin B

All B vitamins are water-soluble substances and therefore any excess is excreted and not stored; thus they need to be replaced continually. The B-complex vitamins are active in providing the body with energy, basically by converting carbohydrates into glucose, which the body burns to produce energy. They are vital in the metabolism of fats and protein. In addition, B vitamins are necessary for normal functioning of the nervous sytem and could well be the single most important factor for health of the nerves.

Nervous individuals and persons working under tension can benefit greatly from taking larger than normal doses of B vitamins, as do cancer patients who undergo chemotherapy or radiotherapy.

Vitamin C

Vitamin C, also known as ascorbic acid, is a water-soluble nutrient, like Vitamin B. Therefore any excess will again be discharged and thus needs regular replacement.

Vitamin C is considered to be the least stable of vitamins and is sensitive to oxygen. Its potency can be lost through exposure to light, heat and air, which stimulate the activity of oxidative enzymes.

A primary function of Vitamin C is maintaining collagen, a protein necessary for the formation of connective tissue in skin, ligaments and bones. Therefore it can be called the mortar of the house. It plays a role in healing wounds and burns because it facilitates the formation of connective tissue in the scar. In addition, Vitamin C fights bacterial infections and reduces the effects on the body of certain allergy-producing substances.

Vitamin D

Vitamin D is a fat soluble vitamin and can be acquired either by ingestion or by exposure to sunlight. It is known as the "sunshine" vitamin because the action of the sun's ultra-violet rays activates a form of cholesterol present in the skin, converting it to Vitamin D. However, too much sunshine is not advisable as it may give rise to metastasis. It aids in the absorption of calcium from the intestinal tract, which is required for bone formation. It helps synthesise those enzymes in the mucous membranes which are involved in the active transport of available calcium.

Vitamin D_2 gives rise to the main cancer suppressor "tumosteron". It is invaluable in maintaining a stable nervous system, normal heart action and normal blood clotting.

Vitamin D is best taken in conjunction with Vitamin A, and fish-liver oils are the best natural source for both these vitamins.

Vitamin E
Vitamin E, a fat-soluble vitamin, plays an essential role in the cellular respiration of all muscles, especially cardiac and skeletal, enabling these muscles and their nerves to function with less oxygen, thereby increasing their endurance and stamina. It aids in bringing nourishment to the cells, strengthening the capillary walls and protecting the red blood cells from destruction by poisons in the blood.

Vitamin E prevents both the pituitary and adrenal hormones from becoming oxidised and because ageing in the cells is due primarily to oxidation, Vitamin E is useful in retarding this process.

This vitamin is also effective in the prevention of elevated scar formation on the body surface and within the body. It protects against the damaging effects of many environmental poisons in the air, water and food. It also has a dramatic effect on the reproductive organs and is often used successfully in the prevention of threatened miscarriages.

I have briefly explained the importance of vitamins, but we must never overlook the fact that vitamins are incapable of performing these tasks without the necessary minerals. The body does not produce the required minerals and therefore these must be obtained from diet.

Minerals are constituents of the bones, teeth, soft tissue, muscle, blood and nerve cells. They are important factors in maintaining physiological processes, strengthening skeletal structures and preserving the vigour of the heart and brain as well as muscle and nerve systems.

Minerals act as catalysts for many biological reactions in the human body. These include muscle response, the transmission of messages through the nervous system, digestion and metabolism or utilisation of nutrients in foods. They are necessary, too, for the production of hormones.

Minerals help to maintain the delicate water balance essential for the proper functioning of mental and physical processes. They keep blood and tissue fluids from becoming either too acid or too alkaline and permit other nutrients to pass into the bloodstream. They also help draw chemical substances in and out of the cells and aid the creation of antibodies.

The body does not require great quantities of minerals, as long as it gets sufficient of the ones that are necessary to ward off illness or disease. Very often an increased intake of minerals can stimulate the cell metabolism and prevent the cell from premature ageing or necrosis, which is dying or decay of tissue.

Some of the essential minerals are as follows:

selenium	zinc
iron	potassium
calcium	chromium
iodine	magnesium
phosphorus	copper

Generally, we will receive sufficient quantities of the required minerals from a normally balanced diet, but as I have said already, in the treatment of cancer and leukaemia these quantities may have to be supplemented. As these minerals are difficult to digest in the organic form, it is better if they are in the chelated form.

Another factor to keep in mind is the presence of sufficient essential amino acids. There are approximately twenty-two amino acids that are the primary components of protein. The following ten are known to be "essential", because they cannot be manufactured by the body independently and must be supplied by foods in the diet:

tryptophane	leucine
lysine	methionine
phenylalanine	isoleucine
valine	threonine
argenine	histidine

Amino acids are necessary to the protein molecule and the quality of the protein is determined by its amino-acid composition. They play a vital role in all physiological functions at the cellular level.

Admittedly, it may take a while for a patient to adapt and respond to a new regime. But it is encouraging to note that most of the patients I know who have taken heed of sound advice today either enjoy good health or, failing that, are able to live a reasonably comfortable life, after having been given a little hope.

Just a few weeks ago I came across a perfect example of this. It concerned a lady who had consulted me in a clinic down south, who had been given very little or no hope for recovery. She had many problems so of course her blood was in very poor condition.

When I saw her recently in my clinic in Scotland, I looked at her and felt obliged to remark on how well she looked. She told me that during her first visit to me she had fully realised how poor a condition she was in. I had asked her then for her promise to follow to the letter the instructions I gave her. She now confirmed that she had indeed done so and therefore could I not witness the outcome!

If the measures I have outlined in this chapter are taken into consideration, they cannot fail but result in restoration of the body. Of course I cannot promise to what degree this improvement will take place. However, the bloodstream will benefit and the acid/alkaline level will be balanced, resulting in a better functioning metabolism and therefore a more effective immune system.

When the body returns to an improved state of health, malignancy will often slow down or regress, because cancer cannot exist in a balanced metabolic system.

You have to believe that disease can be overcome and daily remind yourself of the ways to go about it. Make up your mind to overcome the negative influences on the body so that a good protein balance is obtained — which is crucial in the fight against malignancy — and this will often result in a regression.

Take the general guidelines mentioned into consideration and co-operate with the programme as laid out. This may well vary depending on the individual practitioner, because in alternative medicine there are diverse approaches to cancer treatment. There is, however, no doubt about it that the above guidelines will strengthen the immune system.

To close this chapter I would like to finish with a letter from a patient, which speaks for itself:

"At the beginning of 1978, aged fifty-three, I went to see my doctor (whom I had not visited for ten years) because of increasing fatigue, along with other indications that all was not well with me.

"He immediately decided to give me a thorough examination, which he carried out six weeks later, at the conclusion of which he stated that I had fibroids and would need to see a specialist. Another six weeks later, I visited the gynaecologist, who also gave me an external and internal examination, recording that there was an incomplete emptying of the bladder due to a urine infection, but no disease. I was prescribed more tablets, but given no explanation of the severe pain in my left side.

"Six months after this, I had the first of a number of small lumps with a spot like a boil coming up on various parts of my body. A skin specialist treated me with ointment.

"In the late autumn of 1979, I began bleeding profusely from my bladder, and the subsequent X-rays revealed a tumour within my bladder. For almost two years my strength had been continually ebbing away, so that I was forced to rest a great deal, and the feeling of illness prevailed. I lost three stone.

"My doctor explained to me that unless I had, at least, my bladder removed at once and replaced, I would only live for a short while. Because of a personal aversion towards the description of my future bodily state following the surgeon's major operation, I withdrew, since I felt unable to learn to live with such a thing. Having watched my mother suffer, endure two operations and die of malignant cancer ten years previously, did nothing to inspire faith in this kind of remedy.

"Through friends I heard of Jan de Vries, and flew to Scotland, since I was too weak to travel by road. His kindly manner gave me confidence, and his careful attention and concentration made me hopeful. I began his treatment and followed the special diet, as well as taking the additional natural medicine he recommended.

"Very gradually I stopped going downhill and levelled out. Imperceptibly at first, but definitely, I began to feel a little less ill. Slowly the bleeding stopped altogether and I started to put on weight and get some colour into my face. After one year I commenced taking very short walks, and now walk for an hour each day.

"Everything that Jan de Vries told me to do I carried out to the letter, as one cannot play around with cancer. It is a constant fight. He said to get plenty of fresh air, and this I did, along with deep breathing daily. His suggestion to go into the sea I also managed.

"I ate only organically grown food for two years, despite the monotony caused by the difficulty in obtaining any variety, especially during wintertime, and also drank quantities of beetroot-juice, as instructed by Jan de Vries.

"I certainly do testify to the benefit I have received from this safe method, since I can now accomplish most tasks and live a normal life, with a complete cessation of pain. I thank my

Creator and all those who helped me in so many ways. It is good to be alive. Not only has the condition been obviously arrested, but the growth appears to be shrinking, as there is much less discomfort, more room in my bladder and less movement, too, which I can feel in certain positions. My liver, which was also affected, gives me practically no trouble now, so a return to excellent health seems to be in sight. Sometimes I can hardly believe it has all happened."

5

Organic Germanium

KAZUHIKO ASAI was a remarkable man. I will never forget when, in August 1974 on a beautiful summer evening in Bienne, Switzerland, there was a knock on the door of my hotel room. My stay in this lovely Swiss town was due to my participation in a medical conference. On opening the door I saw an Oriental gentleman who introduced himself in a hoarse voice as Kazuhiko Asai. He immediately impressed me and I invited him in.

We talked at length during that evening and well into the early hours of the morning and that night we established a sincere friendship based on mutual admiration for each other's work, interest and knowledge of natural science. He was totally involved and engrossed in researching the benefits of the mineral germanium to the health of mankind.

We talked that night about our mutual desires and efforts to help alleviate human suffering and it is with great sorrow that I regret Dr Karl Asai (as he is called by his Western friends) cannot now witness the benefits accrued today as a result of his long years of study and research into the properties of this mineral.

He stated that he was neither devoutly religious nor a philosopher, but a researcher of natural sciences. He went on to tell me that at one stage in his life a malignant tumour in his throat had been diagnosed and he let himself be persuaded by his wife to go to Lourdes to seek a cure for this illness.

In fact what happened was that he took the water of Lourdes and his tumour cleared, but his scientific mind was unable to accept that this could be credited to faith alone. He was convinced that other factors played a part and was determined to find a scientifically acceptable answer to the questions which played on his mind. He managed to obtain permission to research samples of the water of Lourdes and, as anticipated, he discovered some remarkable evidence. He was able to confirm the existence of 30 parts per million of germanium in a solution of 10% concentration.

He admitted he had acquiesced to his wife's insistence that he go to Lourdes because around that time he had read some articles which greatly aroused his curiosity. Among these publications were *Journey to Lourdes* and *Man — the Unknown*, both written by Alexis Carrell. He had also read an article which appeared in the magazine *Newsweek*. It was this article that particularly attracted his attention.

The *Newsweek* article was about a three-year-old girl who was dying of cancer. One of her kidneys had been removed, but the cancer had spread to the cranial bones. She had become emaciated, her hair had fallen out and her skin had turned yellow. Her whole system was affected by cancer and the doctors had given her up as a hopeless case. The surgeon at the Sick Children's Hospital in Glasgow, Scotland, recalled that the cancer had spread everywhere. The case had gone beyond surgery and the little girl displayed all the signs of impending death.

As a last resort the child's desperate mother, being a Roman Catholic, decided to take her daughter to the shrine of Our Lady of Lourdes. There the semi-conscious little girl was dipped in the sacred water. The girl, however, was obviously in pain and the pilgrimage was cut short as her mother wanted to get back to Scotland so that her daughter could die at home.

During the first two days after their return the Scottish doctors watched the child slip further towards her death. Then, on the morning of the third day, she sat up in bed and asked for an orange. She seemed to eat this with enjoyment and almost overnight her condition started to improve. Some time later the cancerous tumours disappeared and she once again became a healthy girl.

This story created a major sensation in the medical circles in Scotland and the fame of the miraculous water of Lourdes spread widely. The girl's doctor, a Protestant, insisted that the word "miracle" was indeed suitable on this occasion. The article describing this particular case was featured in the *Newsweek* issue of 9 August 1971 and absolutely fascinated Dr Asai.

He relented under pressure from his family and friends and travelled to Lourdes. After he had been there for a while, he realised a change was taking place and that the tumour in his throat was beginning to shrink. As he was not a zealously religious person, he could not accept that this could be attributed purely to a religious factor. He came to the conclusion that it must be due to something extraordinary in the water of Lourdes, which he was determined to investigate. He transported a quantity of the water to Japan and started his research.

It did not take long to discover that the water of Lourdes contained high quantities of germanium. He was already aware that germanium develops additional oxygen in the bloodstream, so he immediately realised the medical implications of his findings. He wondered if this was the secret of the miraculous water of Lourdes, which over many years has been claimed to have caused dramatic and miraculous cures, or that healing here only took place by faith.

A contributory factor to his determination was the fact that, back in 1945, he had already done some research into this mineral. Towards the end of the Second World War he had been engaged in the task of identifying various samples of Japanese coal for the purpose of petrographical clarification. In those days immediately after the war, no heating was provided. He would pluck tissues from the coal with tweezers, fingers numbed by the cold, and do micro-analysis on the contents of rare-earth elements in each tissue.

Coal is the result of carbonisation of plants that since ancient times have been steeped in seawater due to the sinking of the ground. It is the isolation from air that causes their carbonisation. In petrographical research the following three portions of that black solid coal are distinguished:

—lignin, i.e. stiffening material in the cell walls of woody tissue (in scientists' terms Vitrit);
—mixed clots of twigs, barks and leaves (Clarit);
—clots of seeds and spores (Durit).

The fact that coal contains germanium was already known, but from his examinations Dr Asai concluded that the germanium contained in coal is a primary existent and not a secondary entrant during the process of coal carbonisation. His conclusion did not exactly coincide with the interpretation adhered to by the scientific world at that time, so he was obliged to explain his convictions.

Referring to "living things and metals", he pointed out that in the world of nature, there occurs something akin to metempsychosis (a form of transmigration). Metallic elements in the earth are absorbed by the plants, thus playing a role in their growth. Through plants, animals take in metallic elements, supposedly those transformed into organic metal, which are indispensable for the animal's life. Were this route of transmigration taken otherwise, it would become meaningless.

For example, metallic elements taken in by animals directly from the earth would bring about no effect upon the animal's physical functions. The atomic number of germanium is 32 and this mineral has 32 electrons, which are important for releasing oxygen. It is known that metallic enzymes in living

67

bodies work splendidly in maintaining life. Germanium, by means of its activity as catalyser, in other words through the actions of electrons as explained by quantum mechanics, can enhance the creation of white and red blood corpuscles and at the same time dissolve abnormal cells born inside living bodies.

In 1968 Dr Kazuhiko Asai succeeded in producing water-soluble organic germanium, i.e. when it is dissolved in water the solution remains clear no matter how long it is preserved. This solution, when taken internally, has demonstrated "miraculous" effects on various diseases which are extremely difficult to cure, particularly on tumours. It showed a curative effect similar to that which astonished Alexis Carrell. This explains Dr Asai's interest in the water of Lourdes, because he recognised in it similarities with his solution.

Dr Asai never intended that organic germanium (carboxy-ethyl germanium sesquioxide) be considered a medicine. His view was that it be regarded as an entirely new substance intentionally developed for the sake of mankind. Through its action organic germanium compound is a substance directly related to a living organism. When taken orally, it is absorbed by the blood and so is circulated to all the cells of the body and in the cells oxidation and reduction takes place. Through dehydronisation a large amount of energy-laden oxygen is generated. The organic germanium compound which is bonded with hydrogen is completely discharged from the body in urine and excrement, leaving behind not a single trace.

In his notes Dr Asai states that tests on animals proved that organic germanium compound, after being carried by the blood into all the cells of the body, enters the liver, from there moving to the pancreas, the spleen, the gallbladder and the kidneys before being discharged from the body. Through this process it exerts an effective and appropriate action on the liver, pancreas, gallbladder, kidneys and the suprarenal — as well as the pituitary glands. In addition, it should be noted that organic germanium compound has shown spectacular results on the cerebrum and the cerebellum, which are known to require and consume more oxygen than any other part of the body. The same holds true with the heart.

During our meeting that evening in Switzerland, Dr Asai told me that he had decided to approach me after listening to my afternoon lecture on treatment for multiple sclerosis patients. He was looking for research partners in evaluating germanium in the treatment of cancer, leukaemia and multiple sclerosis, and wondered about co-operation between us in the latter section. I was greatly intrigued by his work and findings and, indeed, a stream of correspondence followed on the subject. Unfortunately, although it was his intention, an opportunity for him to visit our clinic in Scotland never materialised. During the relatively brief time we worked together, however, I learned a great deal from him.

Recently I listened with interest to a medical professor who devoted his lecture to the fact that good health is generally taken for granted. In order to regenerate our cells, they deserve to be treated kindly, which justifies their importance in our physical functions.

Organic germanium effects immediate positive action, which is the supply of additional oxygen to the body cells, giving one energy and a feeling of well-being. After having coursed through the body the germanium will be discharged within approximately twenty-six hours.

Because of increased carbon dioxide in the air — a result of industrialisation and exhaust gases, the gradual reduction in the rain forests and pollution of our oceans and seas (leading to a decrease in plankton) — all human oxygen absorption is under threat. Hence the specific value of germanium in our present environment.

A noted physician once said that giving oxygen to the cells is the best, the ideal, way of curing diseases. Through the discovery of organic germanium by Dr Asai, this possibility has now become a reality.

I greatly enjoyed watching the film "The Water of Life", which deals with Dr Asai's research work into the properties of germanium and was extremely impressed by the positive results obtained from this mineral when used as a therapy.

In his book *Organic Germanium — A Medical Godsend*, which I have studied at length, Dr Asai recalls the words of Schlesinger: "Life is the supreme art created by the hand of a god named quantum mechanics."

In his lecture at that conference in Bienne, Dr Asai told us that he had been charmed by this expression, and increasingly so as his studies in germanium progressed. He regretted that modern science seemed to overlook the importance of this discovery.

However, looking at the current rise to prominence of germanium all over the world, I am sure that Dr Asai would have been more than content. In his own mind the tests which he himself underwent vindicated his beliefs that not only does germanium enrich oxygen supply in the body, it also expels pernicious pollutants from the body, or at least decomposes them to a harmless substance. Oxygen supply is vitally important to our existence and to sustaining life and anything that contributes to a deficiency here can lead to serious problems.

Dr Asai found that adequate quantities of germanium are present in some plants, such as ginseng, aloe, comfrey, chlorella and garlic. Knowing this, we can now understand why these plants and substances are so beneficial to our health.

Although the phenomenon of Lourdes is widely known in the Western world, it is little known that in northern Japan there is also a well of water which has been visited for centuries by people in search of a cure. It has been discovered that the water of this Japanese well also contains a high percentage of germanium.

On a visit to Los Angeles a few years ago, I was told by a colleague that he was about to visit a practitioner who worked with a water obtained from coal reservoirs, as this particular water seemed to have curative effects on the health of people. When this water was researched, it also appeared to contain larger quantities of germanium than usual.

Dr Asai stipulated that during his research work with germanium under atomic no. 32, he had come to recognise the existence of something resembling laws that embrace the natural world but are incomprehensible to man. In his research he witnessed the satisfying results of organic germanium compound on various diseases and at present the possibility is being considered of this mineral being used in the treatment of AIDS.

For more than thirty years Dr Asai devoted most of his time to the research on germanium. Right up to his death he remained involved in this and I remember he once stated that the study of germanium should be conducted on a higher dimensional level than any other types of research. He concluded that germanium was a four-dimensional substance directly connected with life. Semiconductors such as organic germanium play a leading role in the human brain in transmitting messages via the nervous system. He demonstrated that as all organic germanium leaves the body within approximately twenty-six hours it must therefore be supplied continuously in our diet. A deficiency of semiconductors or electrolytes in the brain is supposed to be related to learning disabilities, hyper-activities, failing memories and depressions.

According to Dr Asai, great importance should be attached to the kind of food taken, which should be of the kind that does not cause acidity in the body, as individuals whose blood is acidic will experience a very much delayed healing action. The actual healing process will only start after neutralisation of the blood, thus the intake of organic germanium compound should go hand-in-hand with a careful choice of a proper diet.

Not only is the discovery of germanium as an agent for specific disorders important, but also the knowledge that organic germanium stimulates and strengthens the immune system. It is a highly effective anti-viral agent as it mobilises immune cells to seek out and destroy viruses. The production of interferon, which is a very important "element" amongst the "molecules of the immune system", is also enhanced.

71

In her excellent paper "Germanium, a potent healer", Utah Sandra Goodman stated that the efficacy of germanium is not yet fully appreciated and more substantial clinical evidence is needed in order to properly assess and identify the value of this substance. As a micro-trace element that was virtually unknown, organic germanium and its remarkable therapeutic effects could almost be regarded as an answer to our prayers. I do not doubt that this safe and successful product will prove to be of great value in the future.

In the USA it is said that organic germanium is the elixir of life. Is this really the case or is this an exaggeration?

I am delighted to confirm how often I have seen germanium indeed act as an elixir of life. In quite a few cases I have seen that even small amounts of germanium unlocked the life force within. The amount considered necessary will be decided on by the practitioner and will vary according to the individual patient.

In a report published after research in Japan it is claimed that germanium:

—has the function of inhibiting the multiplication of cells. When this is abnormal it helps to limit the advancement of cancer;
—stops the damage created by radioactivity;
—increases the production of interferon by the body;
—increases the body's ability to absorb calcium from food and supplements;
—subdues the sensation of pain;
—gives increased energy;
—improves heart-muscle tone;
—is effective in removing mercury, cadmium and similar metal poisons from the body.

This last point is worth while remembering when considering the increasing evidence of the damage caused by dental amalgam.

These fascinating facts about germanium hold great future promises for our well-being. By now you will have realised that I am a great admirer of Dr Karl Asai. He displayed tremendous perseverance in his struggle to convince us of the wonderful effects of this now more-or-less recognised product. Therefore I am proud to have been associated with him and for the opportunity to have co-operated with him in attempting to alleviate human suffering.

On my desk I have singled out one of the many letters which I have received from people who have benefited from germanium for all kinds of health problems. This letter, however, concerns the previously serious condition of a five-year-old child with a brain tumour. The girl suffered several epileptic fits a day and after having been given organic germanium compound, the first signs of progress were notice-able in a slight improvement in her speech. Within a week of first taking germanium she was making an effort to walk again and before long she could join her parents on a walkabout at the local shopping centre. Her face had lost its distorted look when she laughed and she had become generally brighter and more cheerful. Her parents wrote proudly that she enjoyed her rocking horse and was able to get about on her little bicycle.

Some of the most comforting experiences with germanium, however, have arisen with people who had clearly come to the end of the road. Those people died peacefully, without pain and with full presence of mind till the very last. Dr Asai's claim that germanium was also a pain reliever has become evident and this wonderful mineral is physically and mentally of great comfort to them.

I remember a young girl who was badly affected by side-effects of the drugs treatment prescribed for lymphatic cancer. When I saw her I immediately agreed with the medical consensus that nothing further could be done for her. She was in great distress and germanium proved to be of significant help to her in the final days of her illness.

On the other hand I am happy to see patients whose lives had been seriously threatened and now share their gratitude that they are still with us thanks to the turnaround germanium effected in their condition.

I often have reason to think back gratefully to that fateful meeting on a summer evening in 1974. I remember that last time I saw Dr Karl Asai, when we said our goodbyes at the little railway station of Bienne, Switzerland. Together with his charming wife, Dr Asai returned to the Far East to continue his valuable work, while my travels took me in the opposite direction.

Thinking of our goodbyes brings back poignant memories. When we shook hands, I felt something pressed into the palm of my hand. He did not relinquish my hand while he said that he wanted to give me a little keepsake. He asked me to promise that I would always carry it in my pocket, because it would give me the energy and the help I needed in looking after my patients. After having given him my promise, I found a small piece of grey-white brittle metal in my hand — a piece of germanium.

6

Enzyme Therapy

THE WORD ENZYME is derived from the Greek word *enzymos* — meaning leavened — and describes a protein-like substance formed in plant and animal cells that acts as an organic catalyst in initiating or speeding-up specific chemical reactions. There are a number of enzymes, but here we are concerned with the prevention of enzyme deficiency. If a lack of enzymes exists, then the chemical processes in the cells are slowed down and altered.

The task of the enzymes is to break down food in the digestive system into simpler substances, which can be more readily absorbed. These enzymes exist in other living things, as well as in the human body. The reaction of our body's life process to enzyme activity is referred to as our metabolism.

Without enzymes many of the essential reactions would not take place. Yet the enzymes which break down the food in the intestines do not endanger the beneficial properties of the ingested food. What they probably do endanger (and I am talking here about the proteolytic enzymes) are body cells making abnormal proteins: cancer cells. They probably are of

75

great value in selectively seeking out these cells and digesting them before they can do any harm.

If the human body was able to produce adequate quantities of proteolytic enzymes, the likelihood of cancer would be minimal. Moreover, proteolytic enzymes have the ability to stimulate the immune system and are also required by the defence system to ward off degenerative cells. Because one of their other characteristics is their ability to prevent the spreading of cancer cells, it becomes obvious that proteolytic enzymes should constitute a major role in cancer therapy.

At his clinic in Mexico, Dr Harold Manner has based his treatment on this particular theory, with which I am very much in agreement, and I have learned much from studying his methods and his motivations. Enzyme therapy should be regarded as a complete integral system to assist in the stimulation of the immune system to detect cancer cells, attack them and hopefully destroy them.

Thus, one factor considered in the treatment of cancer by Dr Manner is the digestive enzyme. In his lectures he claims that cancer is manifested to a great extent by the body's inability to fight off the disease. This results from the underlying factors of inadequate nutrition and the inability of the pancreas and other glands to produce enzymes. Therefore the diet must be supplemented with digestive enzymes whose functions are to aid digestion and, ultimately, through more adequate nutrition, aid the increased absorption of the food ingested.

Various types of digestive enzymes are responsible for the digestion and these are supplied by different types of food. Strict dietary management is not the only essential component of this therapy; Dr Manner also insists that stress decreases the correct functioning of the gastric glands and the pancreas and should be minimised. Therefore these two factors deserve full consideration in any treatment method based on his theory.

For the practitioner it is essential that the action of enzymes is fully understood, as their function is vitally important. Enzymes such as bromelain, lipase, trypsin, chymotrypsin, amylase, papain, pancreatin and many others are important because they are able to act as anti-inflammatory agents, as in arthritis for instance. They can root out several of the major causative factors of inflammatory response and will bring it under control.

Digestive enzymes are essential for the breaking down of proteins, fats and carbohydrates into small molecules, which can be absorbed in the body and give optimal nutrition. We know that nearly all cancer patients have a less than optimal nutrition. It is essential that the enzyme system should be in good working order. This needs attention in all cases of cancer.

It has been jocularly suggested that when, way back, someone dropped a slice of dinosaur meat on to a fire, a turning-point was reached. From then on less care seems to have been taken with regard to nutritional essentials, especially considering our limited ingestion of raw foods nowadays, and our health has suffered because of it. If food is cooked at a temperature of 118°F or higher, any enzymes will be killed. The pancreas, salivary glands, stomach and intestines must come to the rescue and compensate with digestive enzymes to break down the protein, carbohydrates and fats.

Repeatedly, enzymes must be borrowed from other glands and organs and therefore deficiencies elsewhere will occur. The logical conclusion, then, would be to consider that degenerative diseases originate from enzyme deficiencies. In research with different animals it has been proved that cooked food, even when fortified with organic vitamins and minerals, fails to prevent disease.

Raw food immediately releases enzymes and the process of the food being broken down can start instantaneously on ingestion. Fortunately, some areas of current research into cancer are seriously exploring possibilities of finding a cure for this disease with a therapy combining enzyme treatment with supplementary vitamins and minerals. Certainly I have seen some remarkable results where this road has been followed.

The well-known and highly regarded biochemist, G. H. van

Leeuwen, from the Netherlands, has directed a research programme into the characteristics and properties of enzymes which spans many years. It was with great pleasure that I recently had the opportunity to meet this very knowledgeable scientist and I felt that our meeting was most instructive and educational. We discussed at length the advantages for patients when receiving treatment based on carefully monitored enzyme administration.

He informed me that the aim of his research was not primarily to determine the nature of cancer, but was directed towards finding a method for the cure of the disease. All the problems which were not of direct relevance to this purpose have been eliminated as far as possible. The visible course for the complex of symptoms which manifests itself as life, growth and reproduction of the unicellular individual, is now known. Also, the chain of reactions which supplies the energy for these processes, which maintain the cell, was followed. However, with regard to its growth and proliferation, only a number of stimulating or retarding influences are known as yet.

The cell-state is maintained owing to the central control of all its cells, particularly with respect to growth and proliferation. In the organism these cell functions have been completely taken away from the cells, or they are controlled to such an extent that the increase in number and size of all cells is suppressed to within the limits tolerable for this organism. Despite this limited knowledge about the normal growth and proliferation of cells, as well as of their control by the organism, researchers into cancer are trying to find a satisfactory explanation for the abnormal growth and proliferation of one cell of this organism, which has in effect escaped the normal control and which phenomenon manifests itself as cancer.

Mr van Leeuwen maintains that a complete solution to this problem will not be possible before the problems of growth, cell-division and central control, which are allied indissolubly with the phenomenon of cancer, have been elucidated.

The question now arises of whether it is, after all, possible to find a method to destroy the freely growing and dividing cells which have escaped the control of the organism, and to restore this control completely, in other words, to cure cancer.

When we consider how modern medicines, often constituting a specific action on certain diseases, have been developed, we can conclude that the basis for nearly all these medicines has been discovered via the observation of reactions of these materials on the living organisms. By starting from the basic materials thus obtained, further experimenting has resulted in the development of new products.

Only during the last few decades, according to Mr van Leeuwen, have the molecules constituting many of these medicines and their structures been determined, often after lengthy application. Some insight into the nature of the influence of these substances on the organism and on the organisation of the cell-state is only obtained very gradually.

Knowledge concerning the chain of reactions actually occurring in the organism, and in the cells in response to the influence of these substances, is still very limited or even completely lacking. In spite of this, medicines have been developed, in the majority of cases even without any theoretical background, and only based on observations and continual experimenting.

These results prove that medicines can be found exclusively on the basis of observations and deduction without having an exact knowledge of all the reactions and factors which participate in the cure. In principle, this should also apply to cancer.

Mr van Leeuwen, however, claims that cancer is different. As said above, cancer is so closely related to the unknown fundamentals of life, that observation alone has been found to be insufficient to solve this problem. To continue the research effectively, it is essential that hypotheses should be drawn up, i.e. assuming the greatest probability in many factors, and controlled by continual experimentation.

As a result of this work a non-toxic preparation called

Neoblastine was developed by Mr Leeuwen. Neoblastine is a complex of sulphur-metabolising enzymes, which seems to be able to force the illness into regression.

Certainly in our own practice I have been able to witness the benefits of Neoblastine with patients where malignant tumours had been diagnosed. Neoblastine is also mentioned in many publications relating to treatment of gastric cancers in hospitals and clinics. It has also been proved worthwhile as an after-treatment for such conditions.

A recent publication on cancer research featured a special article on research carried out by Mr van Leeuwen. It was claimed that he had discovered Neoblastine. The substance was reported to have shown a favourable effect on the metabolism of cancer patients. In highly concentrated injections it acts directly on the tumour itself and on propagated neoblastic cells. No side-effects to injected Neoblastine were reported.

If patients declare a preference for oral medication I generally recommend that Wobe-mucos tablets or Wobenzym tablets be prescribed, which encourage the absorption process. The Wobe-mucos tablets are made in Germany and contain several kinds of proteolytic enzymes. Compared to other enzyme preparations, the combination in this tablet gives the best results with patients in my experience.

The enzyme combination in Wobe-mucos tablets can dissolve cancer cells selectively in tissue cultures, often apparent through a significant reduction of the metastasis. Patients in the terminal stage of the disease have experienced an improvement in their condition and there is no knowledge of any side-effects to the bone-marrow or to the immune system, nor any risk of haemorrhage.

Even as long as fifty years ago the scientists Freund and Kaminer observed that carcinoma cells are dissolved *in vitro* when treated with the serum of a healthy person. If, on the other hand, serum obtained from a cancer patient was used, cytolysis of the tumour cells did not occur. Christiane and Wolf, independently of each other, established that certain proteolytic enzymes in the serum were responsible for the destruction of malignant cells.

The well-known American scientist, Richard Willstatter, who carried out much research in enzyme substances, was once asked by reporters when a cure for cancer would be discovered. His only response was: "When cancer is cured, it will be by enzyme action."

Each and everyone of us is a product of enzyme action. To make this statement somewhat easier to comprehend, we can read here "enzyme action that controls the metabolism".

In scientific terms human beings should be seen as "dextro" or right-revolving individuals. Cancer is a "laevo" or a left-revolving entity of structure and therefore belongs to the vegetable kingdom, i.e. not revolving to the right. The vegetable kingdom is the oldest and strongest and its enzymes can act right as well as left in the vegetable metabolic process.

Cancer is said to be an extremely complex subject and this is borne out by the extensive research into its origins and to affect a cure for this dreaded disease. It is, however, possible that cancer can be treated when a normal enzyme action of healing is allowed to take place, and indeed I have come across cases where this has occurred.

I remember a gentleman who had the first stages of cancer of the stomach. On evaluation, an absorption problem of digestive enzymes became apparent, mainly due to lack of amino acids, raw glandulars and vitamins. It was totally gratifying to see that the cancer was cured due to the secretion of its own enzyme L-glucosidase. We introduced laetrile amigdalene and as a result the enzyme glucosidase, secreted by the cancer cells, was brought in contact with the substrate laetrile — a cyanide glucocyte — which fractured the L-glucocyte, freeing cyanide gas and destroying the cancerous cells. No damage to the normal cells took place.

With good dietary management and careful administration, this particular patient did very well. This makes us wonder if enzyme deficiency could therefore be one of the possible keys to prevention of this disease.

7

Homoeopathy and Phytotherapy

Homoeopathy
FOR AS LONG as I can remember I seem to have had this childlike belief that if God loves the world, he did not intend it to be populated by sick people. Therefore, when He created the earth He fulfilled the promise that in the field herbs would grow for healing. I also sincerely believe that for every illness nature is able to supply us with a remedy and after practising phytotherapy and homoeopathy for so many years, that belief still exists. I definitely believe that in nature we will find many answers to questions which as yet are still cloaked in mystery.

Everywhere in the world I have seen that different herbs are applied for healing purposes and natural remedies derived from organic matter. The successes thereof have convinced me that although the pharmacopoeias may not indicate these substances as a remedy for serious illnesses such as cancer and leukaemia, these remedies do exist.

First and foremost, of course, we have to endeavour to identify the appropriate substances, after which we have to adapt them for suitable medical or generally beneficial use.

Then it will be up to the practitioner or the specialist to use these in whichever way he or she sees fit, according to the mental picture which has been assembled regarding the patient.

We are greatly indebted to Dr Samuel Hahnemann, generally considered to be the founder of homoeopathy. His four main principles on the treatment of illness or disease are given below.

1. Build up a mental image of the patient as an individual, encompassing body, mind and spirit in this overall picture.

2. Regard disease as a disharmony. Do not attempt to tag a label on symptoms, but set out to discover where the mind, body and spirit are in disharmony.

3. Do not consider medicines as weapons in the battle against disease because, in applying these in order to destroy bacteria, cells and other important matter which are part of our existence will also suffer. Restore the harmony with the aid of harmless, but effective natural remedies.

4. His fourth principle, which I possibly consider the most important in the treatment of cancer, is to remember the patient's own vital force. Will the patient's own defence system be able to stave off infection?

In the treatment of serious diseases the vital force and the strengthening of the defence or immune system of the patient need nurturing and thoughtful care. In this respect homoeopathy comes into its own, considering the whole of the person as an integral entity.

As homoeopathic practitioners, we are sometimes able to classify the characteristics of the patient and with the use of a single homoeopathic remedy, this vital force can be strengthened. Then we will have laid a solid foundation for other remedies we may consider using. This foundation may possibly be achieved by a singular extract or powder, or equally so by a homoeopathic combination. This then could energise that vital force within the body to act as a restorer.

Think of the insignificant little seed and imagine the life force therein when it develops into a large tree. This is something wonderful to behold. So many times in the treatment of serious diseases do we become aware that often insignificant factors, seemingly casually, will change the situation completely. Sometimes the minimum dose of the lowest potency can provoke a reaction which is beyond explanation.

An undetected or unknown miasma, which is a left-over from a former infection, inflammation or virus, may be at the root of all the problems. Yet, that miasma may have been established for generations.

A high temperature may mean a crisis in the body, influenced positively or negatively by the vital force. This force will respond to any sensation in the human body.

I have often seen with cancer patients who suffered from sickness or lack of appetite that Nux Vomica or Centaurium can be of great assistance.

I suspect that the pathologist and bacteriologist Dr Edward Bach realised something of this, which made him turn to homoeopathy before the First World War. He came to understand that the individuality of a person had to be taken account of in any form of treatment. He proceeded to compile certain preparations which became known as the Bach Flower Remedies. Even in minute doses these proved to be of help.

Often with cancer patients we come across a terrifying fear. They do not understand what is happening or know what to expect. Dr Bach studied the characteristics of certain plants and has used rock rose, cherry plum, aspen, red chestnut, and many others in his remedies, sometimes in combination or sometimes alone. His Rescue Remedy is a combination of various natural ingredients which has proved a great help for many a patient.

There are numerous homoeopathic remedies that have a restorative capacity. With these the mental and physical problems of patients can be dealt with. It would take a heavy book to mention all such remedies by name.

These can be related to Hahnemann's four main principles, which have come to be considered the basic laws of homoeopathy:

"Like can be cured by like", or
"*Similia similibus curentur*".

Phytotherapy or herbal medicine

On a recent visit to Hadrian's Wall, not far from Newcastle, I experienced a feeling of admiration when I considered how, so many centuries ago, the Romans had been able to create such an imposing structure.

In the ruins of the foundations of the fortress, I recognised an area which must once have served as a herb garden. In those early days, of course, herbs and plants were necessary for medicinal purposes and were also used for cooking. While sitting there I was thinking about our knowledge of the historical use of herbs, when suddenly I spotted a cluster of unusual plants close by. I thought I recognised this plant, but was surprised to see it growing in that particular area.

To satisfy my curiosity I tasted it and realised that indeed this was the plant which I had come to rely on greatly in the treatment of various ailments, namely the *Petasites officinalis* or butterbur. A preparation based on this plant is frequently prescribed as part of our cancer therapy. I often wonder what we would fall back on if we did not have the use of this plant and its roots.

Alfred Vogel has compiled several remedies based on this plant and I often point out to patients that it serves as a cell renewer. How wonderful to know that plants and herbs exist which have these properties!

When I sit down to have a talk with a cancer patient I sometimes point out that cancer is like warfare. Two armies are fighting each other: on the one side is the army of degenerative cells, and on the other side the army of regenerative cells. If cancer reaches a crisis point, that means that the army of degenerative cells is winning. If we try, however, to make the army of regeneration stronger, with cell renewers such as the above-mentioned *Petasites*, they may be victorious. The fight is always worth while, because I have often seen that cancer has been overcome.

What is this wonderful plant *Petasites* with its powerful action? It is known to have a tremendous influence on swellings and tumours and it can also bring about a change for the better in the cells. Even a single diluted drop of the extract of this plant can effect a change.

Petasan is a Vogel preparation in which *Petasites officinalis* is combined with *Viscum album*. Many times when I have prescribed this remedy, I have seen swelling subside.

I am especially grateful for the availability of this plant when I see younger female patients with complaints about fibroids in the breast. These fibroids can be removed surgically, but can easily recur elsewhere and repeated operations are of course detrimental to one's health, not to mention the trauma that person will be going through every time. Often we have been able to reduce these fibroids in the breast with Petaforce capsules, another Vogel preparation consisting of a concentrated butterbur extract. Also in these cases I usually recommend a high dosage of Vitamin C.

Only recently I saw a young woman who had been advised to have fibroids surgically removed from the womb. She was immediately prescribed this above-mentioned combination and her gynaecologist was astonished by the success. Now similar patients are often informed of this remedy before a decision is made for surgical removal.

It shows the truth in claims that *Petasites officinalis* has been of benefit to mankind for centuries. For a while such remedies were pushed into the background and were superseded by chemical preparations. Thank goodness, though, that we have come to our senses and once again have come to appreciate such effective and harmless remedies.

Cancer patients would do well to take this remedy. When strong concentrations of *Petasites* have been used in the treatment of cancer cases, swellings and tumours have shown a drastic decrease in size, sometimes disappearing totally.

As this plant also acts as an anti-spasmodic, it has been of great help in painful conditions. Not long ago I saw a new patient with serious liver cancer who suffered from a lot of pain. He fortunately derived tremendous benefit from this little plant. Let us not forget, too, that *Petasites* can also be very valuable in the struggle against metastasis. It is not always possible to detect in laboratory research which substance it is in these plants that gives it its effective medicinal properties. For now, let us just accept with gratitude that it does work.

On a fairly recent visit to a university in South Africa, I was told that certain roots, which have been neglected for years, now appear to be beneficial in cancer treatment and full-scale tests to confirm this should be carried out. This makes me wonder if only a small percentage of the billions spent on cancer research was channelled into researching what God has donated to us in nature, perhaps we would have found an effective cure by now. I consider it more important to find a *cure* than to search for evermore for scientifically proven facts about a substance. We need all the help we can find when a patient is in a crisis.

However, it is not just that. How often have we heard it said that prevention is better than cure? Although perhaps there is no such thing as a miracle remedy, we do know that certain remedies have preventive properties. Perhaps when a problem like cancer is detected in its early stages, it can be stopped from developing further by using certain positive remedies.

A number of remedies are known to work excellently when combined with *Petasites officinalis*. The best known of these must be *Viscum album* (mistletoe). Many a time this has proven its valuable properties in the treatment of cancer.

Mistletoe has been the subject of numerous myths and legends. The independent behaviour of this strange, half-parasitic plant suggests something unusual. It needs a tree for its base and with its spherical shape it makes itself a place on the host tree. Centuries back, physicians like Hippocrates and Dioscorides were aware of the beneficial properties of mistletoe and considered it a valuable plant in medicine. Today it is used in cancer therapies the world over.

In the olden days in Germanic mythology the plant was known and it was used by Gaelic priests in their religious services. In folklore many tales have been woven around this evergreen plant.

Back in the nineteenth century Father Kniepp advised the use of mistletoe not only for cramps, circulation problems and epileptic fits, but also for cancer.

Although mysterious tales have circulated about mistletoe, it has been scientifically established that the plant may be used successfully where other remedies have failed.

It is without doubt that mistletoe stimulates the cell metabolism in cases of nervous advanced-age syndrome.

The Druids called it the plant that heals all ills, which may sound like an exaggeration. However, in our clinic I have found that when tablets prescribed for high blood pressure had no success, *Viscum album* proved a useful remedy and this is also true in cases of blood disease and cancer. I honestly would not know where to begin if I had to list the many cases where treatment has included the remedy based on this particular plant and the successes we have witnessed.

This mystical plant with its unique character has been the cause for anthropological practitioners to make *Viscum album* the essential factor in their therapies which are among those described in Chapter 9. Alfred Vogel and I discussed this a few months ago when I visited him in Switzerland. We passed the Ida Wegman's Clinic and talked about the anthroposophical way of treating people with *Viscum album* or, as it is more widely known, Iscador. Both of us agreed on the tremendous results that have been achieved with the Iscador treatment.

Not only from the point of view of strengthening the body's immune system, but also in inflammatory conditions, it has proven of tremendous value in the treatment of cancer patients.

Anthroposophical practitioners often refer to cancer as a "cold" disease. Hence their theory that when using Iscador they aim to warm the vital force or inner spirit by stimulating the thymus gland and thus raising the body temperature. This will increase the number of white cells and antibodies. Therefore it would also seem to be a wonderful remedy in terms of protection or prevention.

The Hahnemann principle of body, mind and spirit is along the same lines as anthroposophical thinking and indeed *Viscum album* is also highly appreciated in homoeopathy.

An unusual case springs to mind of a cold and distant female patient, who showed no emotional feelings at all. She had a nasty, non-malignant swelling on the leg, which would not respond to any treatment. I made up my mind to inject this particular swelling with a mistletoe extract. Initially she became very upset when the swelling increased, reddened and became more painful. After a night of bitter complaints and reproaches, she noticed the next morning that the swelling was largely reduced and the pain had subsided. She suddenly opened up and told me about her inner fears and hidden emotions which she had bottled up for so long, not wanting to confide in anyone.

When she left the clinic after treatment was finished, she remarked that she felt a new person. She had benefited not only physically but felt as if mentally an even greater cure had been effected.

Each time that I have worked with the Iscador preparation, I have always been aware of its tremendous potential. Depending on the case in hand, Iscador can be injected or administered in tablet form.

I remember a young man whom I treated in a clinic in Birmingham. Suffering from an inoperable tumour, he reacted very well to Petasan and Viscasan, together with a vitamin therapy. He is again able to do his work and feels so much better as the tumour is now controlled.

This is an example of some of the happy cases we are involved with. Unfortunately, this is not always the case;

we often come across great disappointments as well. I sometimes point out to patients that I prescribe to the best of my knowledge, but it is only God who cures.

It is often said that herbs are for healing and curing. Despite persistent opposition from some quarters, I insist that herbalism should be regarded as a science, as scientific proof exists as to its effectiveness. The lack of detrimental side-effects in herbalism and homoeopathy and its proven efficiency, makes it a valuable branch of the medical science as a whole.

At a cancer conference I attended and also lectured at on my most recent visit to Canada, it was established that many patients claim to have been cured by Essiac (a Canadian herb mixture) — a treatment which is not yet readily available as further research is still ongoing. The same applies to the South American discoveries based on the lapacho bark, or the medical properties of the creosote bush, which is so highly valued by the Papagos Indians. Claims have also been made as to the medicinal value of Taheebo tea.

These remedies appear to have in common the ability to combat malignant growths, but research for more conclusive evidence still continues. I mention these to show that there are many herbal remedies which could be introduced for the treatment of cancer before too long.

Even going through notes which have been collected by my family over several generations, I have found recipes for tea mixtures that we used for treating swellings and sores.

The old-fashioned remedy of castor-oil — *oleum ricini* — can still play an important role today. Compresses of castor-oil on cancerous swellings can sometimes bring great relief.

It is wonderful to know that the vital force in the human body can be influenced and stimulated by herbs and plants. Hopefully, future research will provide us with further insight and knowledge in this enormously wide field of alternative medicine.

8

Dietary Management

IT WAS A SIGN of great foresight when the eminent scientist Thomas A. Edison stated: "The doctor of the future will give no medicine, but will interest his patients in the care of the human frame, in diet and in the cause and prevention of disease."

Many times in my experience I have found reason to underline this statement. Sometimes in lectures I ask my audience to draw a mental picture. When we set about building a house, we will look around for dependable building materials. We will make sure that we have a sound foundation on which to base a reliable framework. After all, for most of us the biggest investment we ever make in our lives is the house we intend to live in. Nothing about that can be left to chance or taken for granted. Why do we then not apply these same principles to our body and health?

If the roof of our house were to come tumbling down around us, we can have it repaired or move into another dwelling. We cannot apply that to our body as the body we are born with will be the only one we will ever have throughout our lives.

If we relate this building programme to our body we will realise that when the correct building materials are used, i.e. through nutrition, we stand a better chance of leading a healthy life. On top of our house of good health we place our mind or our spirit as an imaginary roof. Hence the saying: *"Mens sana in corpore sano"* — a healthy mind in a healthy body!

Another way of looking at it is that a good roof cannot be supported by a weakened structure. Nor can a sound structure survive on inadequate foundations.

The pillars of our imaginary house rest on some very important factors:

—nutrition
—digestion
—elimination
—circulation
—relaxation.

When these factors are taken care of we can expect a good chemical balance. Health or sickness depend on many influences, such as genetic, environmental, congenital, nutritional, degenerative, psycho-social and atmospherical influences, trauma, bacterial or viral infections.

Of the five listed factors I mentioned earlier, nutrition and digestion take first and second place. When food enters the mouth it makes its way to the stomach and the duodenum. If the absorption is correct, depending on the presence of amino acids, glucose and essential fatty acids, it will be transported to the small intestine, where elimination of residual wastes to the large intestine is to take place. Correct elimination of waste material will benefit our kidneys, lungs and skin. The circulation of the blood will then look after the liver, heart, organs and our cellular system.

Regeneration of our cellular system depends again on amino acids, glucose, essential fatty acids, enzymes, vitamins, minerals and oxygen. If we are to encourage and stimulate the circulation in its vital task, we have to realise that relaxation is essential.

If we look at the framework of the body, or the skeleton, we should realise that to give structure to this, there are some ten trillion cells throughout the body. These, together with body fluids, make up the human body.

Let us not forget, then, that with every tick of the clock cell degeneration occurs, when thousands of cells die. So the cell renewal process is an ever-continuing operation. All these functions depend on the individual pillars being sound and each being given the opportunity to perform their allotted tasks.

If we consider for a moment the importance of looking after this framework with the aid of beneficial regenerative influences, we possibly realise the often overlooked factor of oxygen. This is a major reason for germanium being included in cancer and leukaemia therapies, as discussed in Chapter 5.

We can stimulate the presence of oxygen in the blood, but in order for our body to benefit from this, proper blood circulation is essential. If the circulatory system does not function properly, neither food nor waste products can enter or withdraw from the cells.

Good oxygen transport may be encouraged by relaxation, meditation and visualisation. If the bloodstream is clear, the blood will carry more oxygen and will flow more freely.

Although germanium does improve the oxygen transport, wherever possible let us try and take care of this in our own way. "Tank" your own oxygen. In other words, take physical exercise in the fresh air. Make up your mind to go regularly for brisk walks, as this will enhance the oxygen flow.

A variety of diets have been advocated expressing different approaches to the achievement or maintenance of good health. Admittedly, these can be confusing to the public and for that reason I would advocate that the basic rule should be that food be kept as natural as possible. That is the first and major step on the road of proper dietary management.

It is logical that, for example, a diet to curb high blood pressure is different from a diet designed for a diabetic, or one to enable you to lose weight. This is also the case with a cancer diet. Various cancer specialists have their own different versions, according to their own convictions. If, however, the dietary recommendations from these specialists vary, but generally aim at a good natural food pattern, they all will no doubt fulfil their purpose.

It may seem surprising that the old nutritional and hygiene laws as mentioned in the Old Testament still hold good today. Perhaps this is the explanation for the claim I once read that the Jewish population has a low rate of cancer.

Good nutrition means a balanced diet containing adequate quantities of proteins, carbohydrates, water, fats, vitamins, etc. Chemical additives, artificial flavourings or colourings and preservatives should be avoided wherever possible.

I remember visiting Dr Nolphi's clinic in Sweden some years ago and being very impressed by the treatment cancer patients received there. They were guided and counselled throughout the period of treatment. The diet at that clinic was largely based on ample supplies of fresh vegetables. Although I do not advocate an exclusively vegetarian diet, I will say that if these vegetables are freshly picked and responsibly grown, they will contribute towards a healthy cellular system.

No matter for which purpose I am asked to compile a dietary programme, I admit that one of the rules I will always adhere to is that no pork in any shape or form is included. This means that bacon, pork sausages, ham, etc. are all considered to be out of bounds. Pork contains high animal acids and animal fats, i.e. saturated fats.

Refined sugar and flour, i.e. white sugar and flour, have had all the goodness removed during the "purifying" process. Even polished rice has lost most of its nutritional value.

Coffee, tea or chocolate are of no value whatsoever and there is little or no place for these items in a responsible diet. Instead use herbal teas or Bambu coffee, made from chicory, figs, wheat, barley and acorns. This instant coffee substitute from the Vogel range has a very pleasant aroma and contains no caffeine.

The quality of our drinking water is also important. Oddly enough, we take preventive measures when we go abroad and resort to bottled water. This is to avoid the risk of gastro-enteritis. In our own country the drinking water is responsibly purified and therefore there is no need to resort to these measures. Consider, however, the many regions where additives are supplemented to the water, e.g. fluoride, possibly the most widely known of the additives used in our daily water supply. For this reason it may be worth considering the change to bottled mineral or spring water.

I would also suggest that one considers avoiding the use of aluminium cooking utensils. It is wiser to cook in enamel, glass or stainless steel pots and pans.

Replace salt with Herbamare from the Vogel range. This is a herb seasoning salt containing sea salt, celery leaves, leeks, celery roots, water and garden cress, onions, chives, parsley, lovage, basil, marjoram, rosemary, thyme and kelp. Herbamare is especially nutritious as it is made from fresh, organically grown herbs and unrefined sea salt, plus natural iodine from kelp. Use Herbamare in cooking and at the table.

Avoid chemical preservatives in processed foods, TV dinners and "ready meals", which are generally referred to as "junk foods".

For cancer patients even more than others a good acid/alkaline balance is essential for the existence of all living cells. In my book *Arthritis, Rheumatism and Psoriasis* I have explained the importance of potassium in the maintenance of the pH balance or the acid/alkaline balance. The cellular system requires a high content of potassium. For this reason processed foods are to be avoided, as there is a need in the bloodstream for sodium, calcium and potassium.

A healthy body requires plenty of fluids and a regular intake of mineral or spring water, fruit or vegetable juices is advisable. This will help to cleanse the body and dispose of waste material.

We have to understand that a balanced diet is extremely important for a cancer patient. There is sufficient evidence to suggest that cancer can be caused by a badly managed or deficient diet, certain additives, smoking or drinking. It is important that detoxification takes place before commencing any treatment and during this detoxification period it is better to avoid proteins. This applies particularly to protein foods from animal sources, e.g. lamb, veal, seafood, eggs, beef, pork, milk and milk products. These foods are difficult to digest and will restrict the absorption process.

Pancreatic enzymes digest proteins and these enzymes are part of the immune system especially necessary to resist cancer. Excess protein intake uses up too many enzymes and therefore restricts the enzyme function.

An additional danger with animal proteins is the possibility of residues of preservatives, antibiotics or carcinogenic material. It is better to adhere to foods with a low protein content but which also contain plenty of amino acids which are essential for a good balance. In this category we can include potatoes, alfalfa sprouts, asparagus, beans, beansprouts, beetroot, broccoli, Brussels sprouts, cauliflower, carrots, cucumber, lentils, turnips, tomatoes, seeds (especially sunflower seeds), bananas, nuts and all dried foods.

Animal acids and animal fats are detrimental to health, hence my warning against pork in particular. Smoked or barbecued meats should be excluded and it is much better to use soya products instead.

Some fruit and vegetables are especially rich in proteins, such as apricots, apples, avocados, grapes, olives and tomatoes, and being non-animal protein these are of great value.

The importance of organically grown vegetables becomes clear when we consider that in our own organic nursery we regularly have our soil tested for the presence of minerals and trace elements. These are found in much higher quantities than in soil which has been prepared with artificial fertilisers. Organically grown vegetables inherit this abundance of minerals and trace elements from the soil in which they were grown.

Use vegetables which are as fresh as possible and always

wash and scrub the produce thoroughly before use. Moreover, in order not to destroy the vitamins and enzymes, it is better to eat vegetables fresh and raw, rather than cooked.

It is better not to mix fruit and vegetables and when vegetable or fruit juices are used, please take them separately. It is also important that juices be drunk as soon as possible after being prepared or they may lose their vitamin content. With this knowledge we can understand why the nutritional value of canned or tinned juices is so much less than fresh ones.

Now on to carbohydrates. I have already mentioned the lack of nutrition in white flour and sugar and I consider it better to eliminate these products completely from the programme. Natural sugars, such as honey, molasses, raw and dark-brown sugar or carob products can be used instead. The potassium content of molasses in particular is very high and as a sweetener it is excellent.

For a good balance between carbohydrates and proteins, rice is one of the finest products, capable of balancing the acid/alkaline level. So, let us not forget to include wholegrain brown rice in the diet.

Fibre is most important in any diet, as that is the part of the food that is not digested by the body, such as the skin of an apple and the husk of a wheat kernel. The normal functioning of the intestinal tract depends upon the presence of adequate fibre in the food. That will rule out constipation, which is still a widely experienced problem and, if not the cause, is most definitely a contributory factor in cancer of the bowel or colon. Make sure that the diet contains adequate fibre by including cereals, grains, nuts and oils. Vegetable oils, such as olive-oil, safflower-oil and sunflower-oil are very important. The best sources of fibre, however, are unprocessed grains, such as rice, oats, barley and wheat, which help promote a good cleansing action. Remember, that which was imported needs to be exported within the span of twenty-four hours.

A small pat of butter for spreading is actually less harmful than a poor quality margarine, because margarines are produced by heating the unsaturated fatty acids. Moreover, butter contains more enzymes than margarine, which promote a better absorption. In fact, there exists much misunderstanding on the use of butter and margarine. I know of only one brand of margarine which may be used responsibly and therefore I prefer a scrape of butter instead. The warning against butter based on its cholesterol level, as used in margarine advertisements, is not altogether fair. Butter contains the necessary enzymes for a good breakdown of nutrients.

In order to achieve the necessary detoxification, a fast for a few days could well be advisable. In such circumstances I usually advise that at meal-times either mineral water, fruit juice or at the most a vegetable juice is taken. Here, perhaps it is wise to mention that not all mineral water is good for you. Water is taken for what it can flush out of the body. The best available in this country is Malvern water, in France Volvic water and in my own country, the Netherlands, Spa Blauw. There is so much confusion about tap-water that it is advisable and informative to read the book written by Dr H. C. Moolenburgh, *Fluoride: The Freedom Fight*.

For proper digestion it is also important to accustom ourselves to eat slowly and chew our food thoroughly. Enzymatic action originates in four areas of the body: the salivary glands, the stomach, the pancreas and the wall of the small intestine. Digestion actually begins in the mouth, where chewing breaks large pieces of food into smaller pieces. The salivary glands in the mouth produce saliva that moistens the food in readiness for swallowing. This saliva contains enzymes necessary for the breakdown of the food in preparation for the digestive processes.

Active chemical digestion begins in the middle portion of the stomach, where food is mixed with gastric juices, again containing enzymes.

After several hours the food will have turned into fluid, which is then ready to be transported to the small intestine, where the pancreas will start to secrete its digestive juices.

If fats are present in the food, enzymes produced by the liver and stored in the gall-bladder, will be secreted, breaking the fat into small particles so that it can be broken down by the pancreatic enzymes. The remaining undigested products will enter the large intestine and are eventually disposed of.

Don't you get the feeling when reading about this digestive process which takes place voluntarily and spontaneously, that it can be compared to a well-run factory or laboratory? The one proviso being that the management in charge is aware of its responsibilities.

Something else worth mentioning is that it is considered unwise to drink liquid immediately before or during a meal. Nor should cancer patients take excessively cold or hot foods or drinks.

I have already hinted at the many different dietary approaches available. Maybe one favours a vegan diet or a macrobiotic diet. I will not go into detail on these, as there is plenty of literature available explaining the principles of these dietary regimes.

In this book I prefer to expand on some of the diets which have been designed particularly with the view to controlling cancer or to its prevention.

First of all I would like to start with Dr Vogel's general diet, in other words a diet which is not specifically designed for cancer patients, but rather for general good health.

Dr Vogel's general diet

Breakfast:

Vogel's breakfast muesli mixed with the juice of an orange or grated apple or half a banana or other fruit.

One or two pieces of rye crispbread or wholemeal bread spread with natural vegetable margarine (sunflower- or corn-oil margarine).

One cup of tea after the meal, preferably peppermint, rose-hip or camomile tea. Bambu coffee may be used as an alternative.

Midday meal:
One plate of fresh vegetables, especially carrots and beetroot. The fresh vegetable are mixed with a dressing made from olive- or sunflower-oil with a little lemon juice or celery juice. Baked or steamed potatoes in their jackets may be taken with the vegetables.
For dessert take natural unflavoured yoghurt, with honey if sweetening is necessary.

Evening meal:
Vegetable soup made with fresh organically grown vegetables.
Use salt sparingly in the soup – a little Herbamare is more beneficial.
The soup can be followed by a little muesli and/or a fresh fruit salad. If there is a tendency to indigestion do not combine these two.

General advice:
Animal fat is prohibited.
Use eggs sparingly.
No white flour, or white sugar (or products made with them).
No pork, sausages, bacon or ham.
Cut down as much as possible on coffee, alcohol, nicotine and sweets.
Take plenty of exercise in the fresh air.

I would now like to continue with the diet Alfred Vogel has designed specifically with the new to patients with cancer of the liver, before moving on to some general guidelines which come under the heading of the "New Approaches to Cancer" diet.

Alfred Vogel's liver diet
Recommended foods:
Take only vegetables, especially raw ones.

Salads mixed with Molkosan.
Toasted wholemeal bread, rye crispbread, sunflower- or olive-oil, honey.
Herb tea, apple juice, Molkosan, blackcurrant juice.
Natural brown rice (see below), grapefruit, grapes and berries, buttermilk and low-fat yoghurt.

Foods to be avoided:
Absolutely no coffee, tea, alcohol, white sugar, white flour (and products which contain these ingredients), vinegar, tinned produce, fruit not listed above, meat, fish, butter, fried foods, spices, cucumber, cabbage, cauliflower or spinach.
No sweets or chocolate.

General advice:
Eat twice daily a plate of grated carrots. If possible walk for about an hour to one and a half hours.
Set one day a week aside as a fasting day. During that day take nothing but apple juice, camomile tea and some carrot juice.
Twice each day spend fifteen minutes on breathing exercises.

Recommended preparation method for wholegrain brown rice:
Put rice in a casserole or pyrex dish. Pour boiling milk or water over it and have the oven ready at a high temperature.
Cook the rice for only ten or fifteen minutes.
Switch off the oven, but leave the dish to continue cooking for a further six or seven hours.
Cut up some vegetables such as parsley, chicory, celery and cress and mix these through the rice with a little garlic salt.
Heat up the rice mixture before serving.

New approaches to cancer diet:
Meat and fish:
The digestive system of the cancer patient is severely overtaxed. Because of this it is recommended that all meat is avoided, certainly until the cancer has been halted.
It would seem that chemotherapy affects the body's uptake of protein, so patients undergoing this treatment may feel

101

the need to include animal protein in their diet. This should be taken in the form of non-fried deep-water fish, as this is likely to be the least contaminated. It may be purchased as frozen fish, but should not be flat fish or shellfish as they live in the most polluted regions. Freshwater fish is also not recommended due to high levels of river pollution and mould residue in fish feed. This fish should still be taken only in *strict moderation*.

Fats:
Fat intake should be kept to a minimum and all high-fat foods avoided. In cases of breast cancer *all* dairy products, fats and margarines (including "health" ones) should be kept to an absolute minimum and avoided if at all possible.
For other cancers modest amounts of buttermilk, cheese or yoghurt, made from sheep's or goat's milk, may be included.
When oils are used we recommend the first cold-pressing of organic safflower-, olive- or grapeseed-oil.
When fats are heated carcinogenic substances are produced; therefore this should not be done for cooking purposes. Ghee, olive-oil and grapeseed-oil are preferred, when they are absolutely necessary in recipes.

Vegetables:
Freshly picked vegetables, preferably organically grown ones, are very important. They should be eaten raw, except for potatoes, especially in cases where the cancer is advanced and in all cases early in the treatment. Beetroot is very beneficial.
All vegetables should be well washed and then soaked in water. Potatoes must have all "eyes" removed.
It is suggested that salads are sprayed with a solution made from one teaspoon of Vitamin C powder and 1 litre of water as this reduces the rate of oxidation, thus helping the digestive process.
There is some evidence that parsnips, celery, parsley, mushrooms and green potatoes should be avoided. Tomatoes are only beneficial if eaten directly after picking.
Garlic and onions are both recommended, the former as a

source of germanium. It is best when swallowed in small pieces (with a little water if necessary) before meals. Onions are best eaten raw, mixed with sauerkraut and live yoghurt or other lacto-fermented products.

If onion is to be cooked, it is best to spray it with the Vitamin C solution described above.

A recent survey showed that fruit and vegetables in shops are likely to be contaminated by weedkillers or insecticides. Since such chemicals are poisonous, they should be avoided as far as possible. This can be done by eating organically grown produce (marked OG), which is now becoming more generally available. Grain is also at risk, so try to purchase organically produced flour from wholefood shops.

Grains:

There is some evidence that a gluten-free diet should be followed for three months after the diagnosis of cancer. Rice, millet and buckwheat are to be substituted for other grains.

For anyone interested, a recipe for a delicious sprouted bread is given on page 105.

Nuts:

These should be washed and soaked overnight in a solution of one teaspoon of Vitamin C powder to 1 litre of water.

Unbroken nuts are best and dry-tasting ones are to be rejected. No peanuts should be eaten as they are prone to the development of highly toxic substances.

Fresh and creamed coconut are good food sources.

Legumes and seeds:

These should be sprouted and eaten raw. If cooked, they should be taken in small quantities, well washed, properly cooked and combined in casseroles, soups and salads (not more than four times a week). Brown beans (sometimes known as ful-mesdames) and soya beans should be avoided.

Fruit:

A varied intake of fresh or frozen fruit, preferably in season, is beneficial, but not in excess.

Of the imported fruits, paw-paws, mangoes, kiwis and persimmons are recommended.

Preferably, the fruit should be organically grown, unsprayed, non-irradiated (avocados often are to give them a longer shelf life) and untreated (oranges and pineapples usually are, to enhance their colour). If you wish to follow this advice, ask your supplier to check on these points. Consumer pressure will help change existing practices.

Dried fruits should be washed and soaked overnight in Vitamin C solution. They should not be cooked.

Eggs:

Eggs from free-range, non-antibiotic-fed birds may be used in very limited quantities, i.e. one or two per week, mainly as a method of varying the diet.

There is some evidence that they should be totally excluded in the diet of patients with brain tumours.

Sugar:

No sugar of any sort, including honey, should be used. Occasionally, and as a special treat, a little locally produced honey or very high quality heather or acacia honey may be used.

Water:

The only system capable of removing a high percentage of all foreign substances in water is reverse osmosis, which removes a high percentage of all impurities.

Bottled water is an alternative.

Tea and coffee:

Tea, coffee (including decaffeinated and grain substitutes) and herb teas (unless prescribed) should be avoided.

Purified water and pure, freshly pressed or frozen concentrated juices may be substituted. If this creates difficulties or stress, then one cup of weak tea per day made from Luaka or China tea, if necessary with skimmed milk, may be taken. A herb tea from lime (linden) blossom may also be taken.

Soups made from fresh vegetables may also be used as a drink. In all, patients should consume at least 1 litre of fluid per day.

Salt:
No salt should be used. Herbs like hyssop may be used in soups and cooking as flavour enhancers.

Alcohol:
Whilst a little alcohol such as one glass of red wine with a main meal is permissible, all neat spirits should be avoided. Cheap wines are often contaminated with suspect chemicals and their processing is questionable. Wine from organically grown, non-sprayed vines, is available and is grown by the Lemaire-Boucher method. Some major wine shops do stock these products and it is worth while knowing that they are identified as such on the label.

Preparation of unyeasted sprout bread:
This "simplest of breads" contains only sprouted wheat: nothing else. The commercial versions sold under the brand names Essene and Wayfarer's Bread (and perhaps others) have proved very popular, but making them at home is pretty challenging. However, this recipe does work.

If the result of your first try is not successful in some way, either bland-tasting or else too wet, next time pay more attention to the timing of the sprouts, because that is the crux of it. The finished bread should be moist, flaky, dark and a little sweet — dense without being heavy. Its devotees consider it the purest of breads, and since it contains no flour, no yeast, no salt, sweetener, fat, or dairy products, who can argue?

Use about one pound of wheat per loaf. Start with two to three pounds, about six cups of wheat: that will make three good-sized loaves. Choose hard spring or winter wheat. Soak it in warm (room temperature) water for eighteen hours, then keep it covered in a dark place, rinsing it three times a day until the little sprout is one-third the length of the grain. This will take about thirty-six to forty-eight hours maximum. If you fear that the sprouts may grow too long before you are able to have time to grind them up, slow the process down by putting them in the refrigerator towards the end of the time.

If the sprouts are too young, the bread will not be sweet. If they are too old, the bread will be gooey and will never dry out.

Remove the excess moisture from the sprouts by patting them with a terry towel. Grind them with a Corona-type mill or liquidiser, or about two cups at a time in the food processor, using the regular steel blade. Make them as smooth as possible.

What results from the grinding process is sticky, but knead it very well, nevertheless. For this, mechanical help is necessary and if you grind the sprouts in your food processor, just keep processing each two cups for about three minutes in all, stopping just before the doughball falls apart. How long this takes will depend on the kind of wheat you use: watch carefully.

Knead by hand or with a dough hook until the gluten is developed, somewhat longer than you would do with a normal dough. If you are kneading by hand, keep the dough in a bowl and use a hefty wooden spoon or dough knob, unless you want to abandon yourself to the ancient mud-pie method of squeezing it between your fingers until the gluten gets going and the kneading becomes easier.

Whatever method you have used to get to this point, cover the dough and let it rest for a couple of hours or so, then shape it into smallish oblong loaves and place on a well-greased baking sheet.

Bake slowly, not over 125°F, for two-and-a-half hours or until nicely browned. (The bread does well in a solar oven, if you have one.)

Cool the loaves and wrap them in a towel. Put them in brown paper or greaseproof paper bags and set aside in a cool place or in the refrigerator for a day or two. This softens the leathery crust and enables the insides to gain their moist flaky perfection.

This recipe can be varied by the addition of dried fruit. For example, grind half a cup of dates along with each pound of sprouted wheat. Other dried fruits can work well, too, but we like dates best by far. Raisins make a very sticky and black loaf, which is also too sweet unless you reduce the measure by half.

Further advice:

Avoid:　　—roasted, fried or burnt food;

　　　　　—tinned and smoked food;

　　　　　—aluminium cooking utensils and aluminium foil to wrap food in;

　　　　　—cling-film coming into contact with food, as the coating on most brands is carcinogenic;

　　　　　—smoking or smoky atmospheres.

Shop-bought foods should be checked for additives. Try to select foods that do not need preservatives, flavourings, etc.

All foods should be well chewed and prepared and eaten in a peaceful and relaxed atmosphere. Rest or unhurried activity, both before and after eating, enables better digestion.

Laughter and good humour in large quantities is highly recommended.

The Moerman diet

Dr Cornelis Moerman started his career as a general practitioner, but has spent decades on cancer research. Ever since 1940 he has worked successfully with a diet, for which he gives the following basic principles:

—No meat or fish.

—No water, coffee or tea.

—No sugar and only moderate salt.

—Daily ½-1 litre of buttermilk, or porridge made from buttermilk.

—Juice of lemons, oranges and currants.

—Egg yolks (but no whites).

—Wholegrain bread with butter and cheese.

—No potatoes, but brown rice with butter and green vegetables.

107

—Especially salads with cucumbers and tomatoes, also other vegetables such as carrots are permitted.
—Rice cooked in buttermilk.
—Plums, apricots, apple sauce, pears and peaches.
—Pea soup with onions, carrots and vegetables, but without meat or bacon.
—Honey.
—Olive-oil.
—Many fruits, especially grapes.

The diet, as part of a total therapy, is designed to promote general health, because Dr Moerman maintains that cancer is not a local illness, but a disease of the whole of the body. A healthy body will be able to increase immunity against cancer cells. To this end a well-functioning metabolism is needed. This is within our reach if all organs and especially the bowels function properly. To that effect the intestines produce an acid that is able to destroy cancer cells.

Ingested food should not tax the organs, nor should it contain matter which could encourage the tumour. No detrimental matter should be present in the system. For this reason I feel it is useful to include Dr Moerman's more detailed guidelines.

Foods to be avoided
White flour products:
These products have been robbed of most of the vitamins of the B-complex which were present in the skins of grain, and of Vitamin E from the germs. The bran has also been removed, which is important for the discharge of waste matter by way of the bowels. Often harmful fats and other matter have been added (even bleaching agents).

Sugar:
Refined white sugar promotes the growth of tumours and contains no goodness. After the refining process there is no nutritional value left, no vitamins or minerals, and it taxes the pancreas unnecessarily. Fructose or sugar substitutes (artificial sweeteners) should also be eliminated from the diet.

Meat:
There is no place for meat in the diet of cancer patients. Often they are unable to properly digest meat, due to insufficient stomach acids and decay could cause problems. Meat also contains substances that do not belong there, but have been introduced during the breeding process. Resulting from the consumption of meat, detrimental uric acid is stored in the body, which is difficult to dispose of. When a tumour breaks up, extra uric acid circulates in the body.

Fish:
Although fish is more readily digestible than meats, unless it contains excess fats, nowadays many fish contain toxic substances, amongst them mercury.

Animal fats:
These are mostly used after having been heated during the manufacturing process and will then contain carcinogenic substances. Even everyday cooking oil is manufactured by way of a heating process.

Artificial colourings and appetisers:
Many of these have been proven to be carcinogenic and sufficient doubt exists about the remainder of them to suggest that it is wise to avoid them altogether.

Coffee and other beverages:
Not only does it contain caffeine, but during the roasting process more harmful substances are released. For the same reason any roasted coffee substitutes are not allowed. Tea and cocoa also contain harmful substances and neither are herb teas permitted.

Yoghurt:
Yoghurt usually contains sinistral lactic acid, which is not advantageous in the battle against cancer. Moreover, yoghurt destroys non-harmful and necessary bacteria in the large intestine. Biogarde and Kefir natural yoghurts are, however, good for the body as they contain dextro lactic acid.

Tinned vegetables:
These often contain preservatives, which should be avoided.

Legumes:
With the exception of green peas, these should be avoided.

Potatoes:
These mainly serve as a staple food and contain only a few minerals. Besides, the starch from the potatoes is more difficult to separate than other starches. The digestion of this overtaxes the pancreas.

Fried or roasted foods:
These contain carcinogenic substances. The more often oil is reheated, the more damaging it becomes.

Margarine:
All margarines, even those based on vegetable oils, have to undergo a heating process during manufacture.

Rye-bread or pumpernickel:
These often contain anti-mould substances. It is thought that stale white bread is sometimes used up in the manufacture of pumpernickel.

Salt:
Do not use salt unless it is considered absolutely necessary. The cancer cells already contain too much sodium. This rule also applies to sea salt, even though that contains more minerals.

Alcohol:
All alcohol has a harmful effect on the membrane of the cells and is detrimental to the liver.

Smoking:
Smoking should be totally banned.

Permitted and recommended foods
Buttermilk:
Contains dextro lactic acid, beneficial for bowel movement.

Egg yolks:
When eaten raw these contain lecithin, which is destroyed in the cooking process. Lecithin keeps the cholesterol fluid. Choline is very important for the liver. The egg yolk contains many essentials, among them the B vitamins, and is therefore instrumental to good health. The egg whites contain a protein which is hard to digest and which destroys vitamins. Patients with liver or gall-bladder problems, however, should be very wary of egg yolks.

Citrus fruits and lemons:
Here it is that the Vitamin C content counts.

Beetroot juice:
This detoxifies the blood and is especially useful in counter-acting the effects of radiation or chemotherapy. It also promotes the increase of white and red blood corpuscles. Beetroot also has a favourable influence on the liver and gall-bladder.

Brown rice:
The skins contain essential B vitamins. Rice is one of the very few foods that contain all ten essential amino acids, which are necessary nutrients for the body. Organs are reinforced by brown rice, which in turn demands no effort from the organs.

Green peas:
Green peas (not split peas) are important because of the benefits obtained from the proteins they contain. Use in soups combined with other vegetables.

Wholemeal bread:
This contains all the natural nutrients of wheat.

Butter:
Butter does not have to undergo a heating process during manufacture.

Cheese:
If possible choose a cheese in which no artificial colourings

111

have been used, preferably one made with natural rennet and a low salt content. Refrain from eating mature cheeses.

Cereals:
Cereals are mostly acidic and after soaking they can be eaten raw.

Raw vegetables:
If possible use organically grown vegetables. Vegetables contain many valuable nutrients. If these are used in sufficient quantities, cooked vegetables may be omitted. Frozen vegetables may be used, but in limited quantities.

Cold-pressed oils:
Olive-oil and sunflowerseed-oil are rich in Vitamin F, poly-unsaturated fatty acids. However, they should not be heated.

Fruit and fruit juices:
These should not contain added fructose. The fructose that is present in the fruit is accompanied by vitamins and minerals.

Milky puddings:
If possible, use fresh, untreated milk with barley flakes, oat flakes, wheat flakes, rice, etc.

Additional general recommendations:
Always eat slowly and chew thoroughly so that even liquid food is mixed properly with saliva.
Only use water in the *preparation* of food as it does not contain any nutrients. Only the cancer cell would benefit, so it would cause adverse effects.
Use undamaged enamel cookware.
Do not use synthetic washing-up liquids.
Beware of fluoride preparations.
If the crust of the bread is burnt, do remove it.
Spinach may only be used if it has not been sprayed. Any leftovers of spinach should be disposed of as, within a few hours of it having been cooked, harmful substances begin to develop.
Do not store a partly used onion as this attracts harmful bacteria.

112

Dried fruits should be soaked for 24 hours, after which the water should be discarded.

One teaspoon of pure honey is allowed daily.

The last diet I will mention here is my own diet, which can be tailored to suit the individual, as religious, cultural and personal characteristics and preferences should be taken into account.

Diet for the prevention of cancer and leukaemia
Breakfast:
Unsweetened fruit juices (especially pineapple); or fresh fruit – grapefruit, grapes or apple or other fruit; or compote of various stewed fruits with or without yoghurt.
Cereal: All bran or oats – moistened with soya milk or date juice or diluted apple juice or water. Molasses can be added for sweetening. Cereal can be delicious with stewed prunes and their juice.
Brown rice with soya sauce.
Two rye crispbreads or wholemeal toast (take this two or three times per week). Vogel mixed grain bread is also very beneficial.

Beverages:
One cup of tea or instant Bambu coffee per day (without milk or sugar)
Herb teas are beneficial. Choose from rosehip, elderflower, lemon verbena, peppermint, lime blossom, camomile (also Jan de Vries 100% Herbal Health Tea).
Drink diluted fruit juices and/or bottled spring water.

Lunch:
Have a salad every day, especially if it contains raw grated beetroot and carrot. For choice add nuts, cottage cheese, avocado pear, bean and seed sprouts, olives or fruit.
Baked potatoes or brown rice or any whole grains.
Soup made with organically grown vegetables.
One slice of wholemeal bread with possibly some homemade jam.

Dinner:
Lamb – once or twice a week.
Beef – once a week.
Poultry or rabbit – two or three times a week.
Fish (sea/freshwater) – three or four times a week.
Pulses – soya (or tofu), aduki, broad, kidney or haricot beans,
or chickpeas or blackeyed peas – three or four times a week.
At least one day per week have only grains, vegetables and fruit.
Eggs should be limited to a maximum of three or four a week.

Seasonings:
Dress salads with Molkosan, cider vinegar, olive oil or a
combination of olive oil and lemon juice.
Use plenty of fresh herbs, especially parsley, sage, rosemary
and thyme.

Foods to be avoided:
Chocolate, sweets, cheese, anything from the pig, white flour,
animal fat, smoked or pickled food, coffee (except Bambu),
artificial colourings, and certain preservatives and additives,
carbonated beverages and alcohol.

Let me state finally that for any diet to be successful, there
should be total trust and co-operation between the patient and
the practitioner. In fact, that applies to any treatment therapy.
The following advice is also useful.

–To help good digestion take plenty of rest.
–Do not get overtired.
–Make sure to take outdoor exercise for a good oxygen flow.
–Remain optimistic and never forget that it takes many
muscles to frown, but only a few to smile.
–Do not hesitate to ask friends and family for their full
co-operation.

Keep in mind the useful advice from Dr Ann Wigmore,
founder and director of the Research Institute for Useful
Living: 'It is not the food in your life that brings health, it is the
life in your food that really counts.'

114

9

Complementary Therapies

THE MANY ALTERNATIVE cancer therapies available today express the personal views of the doctors and practitioners by whom they have been designed. As I cannot possibly deal with all of them, I will concentrate on the ones I have been involved with myself. In other words, those therapies which I have studied myself in the clinics where they were practiced or those I have studied and applied to our own patients.

The differences between the approaches do not take anything away from the fact that the appropriate practitioner accepts the responsibility for that patient's health and will do his or her utmost to ease the suffering and look for a method to control the problem.

There are methods which have proved their worth in diverse situations and others which have been seen to be effective in a more singular application. Each patient deserves the practitioner's single-minded attention, effort and an open-minded attitude to his or her specific problem.

Sometimes even a minor adaptation in an established

treatment approach has signalled a change for the better in a patient's condition.

I have studied many methods over the years and will discuss only a few in this chapter, but I hasten to point out again that these are by no means the only methods.

First, I would look at the approach of Alfred Vogel from Switzerland, my teacher and mentor for so many years in both homoeopathy and naturopathy. In his recent book on cancer he lucidly and sensibly explains his views on cancer, how it should be approached, the values of diet and the use of homoeopathic and herbal remedies.

His homoeopathic remedies such as Petaforce, Petasan, Milk Thistle Complex, Echinaforce, and many more in the Bioforce range, have shown themselves to be invaluable in the work in our clinic. These remedies have often brought about a change in the condition of patients; *Petasites officinalis* in particular, as a cell renewer in the treatment of cancer, is extremely beneficial. That is the reason the cover of this book features this plant.

Now I move to the work of Dr Josef Issels, who used 'whole body' therapy at the Ringberg Klinik in West Germany. Over the years I have attended quite a few seminars in which Dr Issels was involved and I have learned much from his theories. His therapy is based on the evidence that a healthy body cannot develop cancer, so he treats the whole body with any therapy which might help to build up the body's defences.

Dr Issels believes that cancer is caused by the lack of one or more nutrients, which makes the body deteriorate and causes damaged cells. In a sick body, a condition is present in which cancer can develop. This condition he calls the 'tumour milieu'.

His therapy consists of surgery if possible, radiation if surgery is not possible and immunotherapy in all cases. The strongest emphasis, however, is placed on improving the body's defence system by diet.

Dr Issels maintains that the three main principles of cancer are as follows:

1. Cancer is not a localised disease, but a chronic, degenerative disease of the whole body. Before a tumour can grow, the body must be sick.

2. Cells that can change to cancer exist in every person. When the cancer develops, the body's defences are too weak to resist the change to cancer cells.

3. Tumours are a late stage in the disease. For a cure of cancer the body's natural defence system must be restored.

Similar ideas, but possibly at a more advanced level, are held by another person whom I hold in great esteem. Whenever I turn to him for advice, I always find him co-operative and supportive. Dr H.C. Moolenburgh from Haarlem, the Netherlands, is a specialist in the field of complementary medicine and has spent many years involved in cancer research.

His summary is that the orthodox way of thinking about cancer starts with a degenerating cell. Emphasis is placed on *why* the cell degenerates (carcinogens, oncogens, viruses, etc.) and *how* it degenerates (research in chromosomes).

The so-called alternative way of thinking, which a well-known homoeopath, Dr Piet Kleinepier from Goes in the Netherlands, prefers to call a regenerative theory, starts with a body that, for some reason or another, tolerates the multiplication of degenerative cells. It stresses the point that our body supports a survey system that deals with dangerous situations. These can come from without (bacterial) attack, virus, intoxication, trauma) or from within (cancer being one possibility).

Which analysis is right?

Neither theory is based on rock-solid facts. Both of them are no more or less than belief systems. Why a belief system gains prominence for some time remains a mystery to Dr Moolenburgh. According to him it may have something to do with a vague concept like the 'time spirit'. It is also a fact that belief systems change as times change. The sooner it can be agreed upon that orthodox and regenerative ways of thinking about cancer are philosophical concepts and not two systems, where one happens to be right and therefore the other must be wrong, the better.

He has deliberately chosen the immune concept as it seems to cover most facts and nothing appears to have been omitted. He is, however, quite aware of the possibility that the immune system is part of an even bigger 'thing' that cannot yet be described in exact terms. He considers that this bigger 'entry' may have something to do with people being healed spontaneously from cancer at revival meetings or after a life-altering experience.

Our friendship goes back many years and although we are both very busy with our practices and live in different countries, we manage to stay in regular touch, mostly by telephone. We are, for example, both fervent supporters of the use of mineral germanium in cancer treatment and have discussed the pros and cons of this mineral according to our respective experiences with patients.

Although Dr Moolenburgh has a sound foundation in orthodox medicine, this does not hinder him in his appreciation of alternative approaches, which he usually refers to as 'the gentle approach'.

It seems a long time ago that I first heard of the Moerman Therapy, which I will describe next. Dr Cornelis Moerman, now in his nineties, was involved in cancer research even before the Second World War.

As a youngster Dr Moerman owned carrier pigeons, which he used to enjoy enormously. Not long after he started as a general practitioner in Vlaardingen, the Netherlands, a young lad asked his advice on a sick pigeon. Dr Moerman was told that the boy's father had had the pigeon checked over and it was diagnosed that the bird was suffering from cancer. He now wondered if the doctor could give him any advice. This pigeon set Dr Moerman on the road to cancer research. With a syringe he removed some cancerous cells from the tumour and injected these into the chest muscle of a healthy pigeon. The sick pigeon died after a few weeks, but the healthy pigeon remained healthy. He discovered similarities in the metabolism of pigeons in relation to human beings and over the years has come to the following conclusions:

> 1. The high oxidation capacity of pigeons is influenced by the range of food matters that protect these birds against cancer. Therefore specific elements in food could be an important weapon in our fight against cancer.
> 2. The fact that an unhealthy situation has to be present for a cancer to develop gives reason to believe that cancer could be fought with a similar method, i.e. treatment of the whole person through selected food elements.
> 3. Cancer arises as a result of an unsettlement in the metabolism, namely a decreased oxygenation capacity and an increase in the fermentation process, causing demolition of sugars and carbohydrates, thus producing lactic acid. In other words, when cancer arises, it occurs in an internal organ with a decreased capacity for oxidation, combined with fermentation.

The conclusion is that by taking away the basis, by means of the selected food elements, then there is the chance that cancer may disappear.

For nearly fifty years Dr Moerman has centred his research into cancer on dietary management and as a result he has recognised the role vitamins and minerals perform in the search for an effective cancer therapy.

I was very pleased to learn that the Dutch Institute for Cancer

119

Research has been given an extra grant by the Dutch government for extensive research of the Moerman Therapy. In the meantime, there are already dozens of doctors throughout the country who have adopted his methods over the years.

It is sometimes claimed that the Moerman dietary management is restrictive, but one patient told me that for her it was no longer a mere diet, it was now her life. Certainly, her condition was proof that the philosophy of Dr Cornelis Moerman can be interpreted into an effective therapy.

Recently I was approached by a well-known medical specialist who asked me for further information on the Moerman Therapy. He was very impressed with the remarkable improvement in the condition of one of his theatre sisters and wanted to know more about the background and motivations behind the diet.

Although at times Dr Moerman has been ridiculed by his critics for his unorthodox views, one of the benefits of his methods must be that everyone can afford to follow his advice, because no extra cost is involved in his dietary regime. It would take a large volume to describe the many case histories of patients' improvements with the Moerman Therapy.

Now I come to the work of Dr Ernesto Contreras, a former pathologist with extensive orthodox medical knowledge, who has kindly consented to write the foreword to this book. In his clinic in Tijuana, Mexico, Dr Conteras used metabolic therapy, which includes laetrile, vitamins, minerals and enzymes, with DMSO and live-cell therapy also available. He also uses low-dosage chemotherapy, radiation, and limited surgery, as do most of the European clinics. Dr Conteras has been treating cancer patients with non-toxic therapy for nearly twenty years.

Experiences have convinced Dr Contreras that laetrile can be used for prevention of cancer, and it should be used especially in high-risk situations such as the following:

–if families have one or more cancer patients;
–if families have poor nutrition;

–if individuals work in a cancer-prone industry or environment;
–if individuals suffer from stress they cannot handle.

Dr Contreras recommends that people eliminate obvious stress situations, eat a good diet and take at least one tablet of laetrile a day together with enzymes, vitamins and minerals. This programme should prevent cancer. If a person gets sick, he or she needs extra vitamins, minerals and enzymes. Cancer patients need more vitamins and minerals than non-cancer patients, because cancer is a parasite and steals nutrients from normal tissue. Vitamins A and C should be taken in large quantities.

Any substance that is foreign to the body, such as radiation and chemotherapy, is poisonous and the body cannot tolerate it. Sooner or later toxic therapy will kill the patient. However, laetrile and enzymes have sometimes reduced the toxicity of chemotherapy 100 per cent. Children who have leukaemia can tolerate drugs no longer than three years, which is the total length of time a child can be treated with drugs.

Laetrile and enzymes can and should be continued indefinitely, according to Dr Contreras. After five years the doses can be cut down to smaller amounts of enzymes and vitamins and to possibly one tablet of laetrile a day. But he advises that the dosage should never be withdrawn completely.

It is with fond memories that I recall the times we have lectured together in Canada. And then I remember a patient of his who shared the platform on one occasion and told the audience of how she had approached Dr Contreras at his clinic in Mexico when she had been left without any hope of survival. Yet now she was there on the platform with him!

Dr Contreras has shown many times over that alternative approaches to cancer do work. He spent some time with us in our clinic in Scotland and I have learned a great deal from him. I regard him highly as a colleague and a friend.

This brings me to Dr Harold Manner, PhD, formerly in charge

121

of the Biology Department of Loyola University, Chicago. He now heads his own organisation called the Metabolic Research Foundation. Here cancer patients and other interested persons may call or write in order to obtain the names of nutrition-minded physicians who use the Manner Therapy.

Manner's Metabolic Research Foundation is a non-profit-making organisation, founded to promote research and to disseminate information about cancer and other degenerative diseases. There are more than 150 medical facilities in the United States where health professionals use Dr Manner's methods of treatment.

Dr Manner's metabolic cancer therapy works towards the following objectives:

–maintaining a satisfactory lifestyle;
–a feeling of well-being;
–adequate weight control;
–physical activity;
–good appetite;
–normal skin colour;
–freedom from pain;
–a healthy mental outlook;
–a desire to live a long life.

Diet is the most important part of the plan. High animal protein, high fat and highly processed foods must be avoided. Man primarily has the jaws and teeth needed by vegetarians, not by carnivorous creatures. When a high animal protein diet is eaten, most of the body's enzymes are used to digest the protein, and there are not enough left to digest disease-bearing organisms always present in the body. Meat contains waste products of metabolism, and when a person eats animal produce he will assimilate these waste products. Studies have shown Dr Manner that vegetarian athletes who eat more plant proteins than animal proteins exhibit more than twice the endurance of meat-eaters.

His cancer therapy is based on the use of laetrile with added vitamins A and C and digestive enzymes. He has conferred with physicians all over the world and his therapies are widely used and accepted. The importance of Dr Manner's work is undeniable and research is being continuously maintained.

Dr Max Gerson may be called the father of the 'whole-body' treatment of cancer. Dr Albert Schweitzer called him 'one of the most eminent scientists in medical history'. Since his death in 1959 his work has been continued by his daughter, Charlotte Gerson Strauss, at her clinic in Mexico. She has visited the United Kingdom and given several lectures explaining her father's theories on cancer treatment.

She underlines his ideas that a normally healthy body can keep all cells functioning well. Abnormal growths and changes are thus prevented. It follows, therefore, that if the body can be returned to normal, cancer can be prevented or controlled. Dr Gerson emphasised that cellular energy is obtained with the use of oxygen in healthy cells, but without oxygen in cancerous cells. The malignancies in cancer patients go deeper and deeper into the non-oxygen energy. Thus the body becomes more poisoned and has less defence against disease.

The inflammatory process in cancer patients is weak and the body cannot make white blood cells to heal infections. If the immune process is strengthened by non-toxic therapy, it may then be able to fight infection.

Dr Gerson advocated that we must:

1. detoxify the whole body;
2. provide essential minerals of the potassium group;
3. add enzymes in the form of green leaf juice and fresh calf-liver juice.

This treatment will allow the oxygen energy cycle to function, but the cancer cells will not be able to adapt to it, so they will die.

In his book *A Cancer Therapy*, Dr Max Gerson pointed out

that when cancer reaches an advanced stage, almost all the organs will be involved, especially the liver. All the necessary elements have to be present to help in its prevention and control: vitamins work with enzymes and enzymes work with hormones and minerals.

Cancer develops in a body that has lost varying degrees of its normal function because of a poisoned liver. The poisons originate from chemicals present in air, food and water, as well as from nutritional deficiencies, which poison cells. One of Dr Gerson's recommendations, therefore, is that where possible we must eat natural foods, grown organically.

His regime for cancer patients is very strict. It is designed to rejuvenate the liver, the largest single organ in the body. The liver can be damaged for a long time before it shows any signs, because it has many stored reserves. The liver has numerous functions, most of them combined with functions of other organs. It is so unique that it is sometimes called the 'balance wheel of life'.

Dr Gerson's therapy can be applied to conditions other than cancer, such as:

–toxification during pregnancy;
–turberculosis of the lungs and other organs;
–arthritis deformans in advanced stages;
–mental diseases and bodily weaknesses;
–spastic conditions, especially angina pectoris.

In order to feel better more quickly, patients are encouraged to take coffee enemas to eliminate toxins and strengthen the live, or so that it can change starch into energy and help prepare the body to use the oxygen energy pathway. These should be given every four hours at first, day and night, even more frequently if pain is experienced. For this purpose it is advised to use two tablespoons of ground coffee beans infused in half a litre of water. It is wise to take high dosages of vitamin C during this period.

Every other day two tablespoons of castor-oil are taken by mouth, followed by a cup of black coffee, and five hours later, a castor-oil enemas, in addition to the coffee enemas.

Large amounts of peppermint tea taken by mouth will help wash out the bile from the stomach and make the patient feel better. Coffee is not taken by mouth except to help eliminate the castor oil from the stomach by stimulating peristalsis.

Proving his insight, Dr Gerson has stated: 'Everybody has a healing mechanism – the doctor's role is to activate that.'

As Dr Gerson advocates the use of castor oil in his therapy, this may be an opportune time to mention that I recently saw a weeping carcinogenic wound that was cured with the use of a castor-oil pack. I know that my grandmother and great-grandmother were very much in favour of this treatment method and for the reader's benefit I will give you Dr Edgar Cayce's instructions for this purpose:

Material needed for castor-oil packs:
Flannel cloth
Plastic sheet (medium thickness)
Electric heating pad
Bath towel
Two safety pins

Instructions:
First prepare a soft flannel cloth (preferably wool flannel, but cotton flannel can be used if this is not available), which measures about ten inches in width and 12 to 14 inches in length after it is folded to two or four layers. This is the size needed for abdominal application; other areas may need a different size pack as appropriate. Pour some castor oil on to the cloth. This is done without soiling if the plastic sheet is placed underneath. Make sure the cloth is wet but not dripping with the castor oil. Then apply the cloth to the area which needs treatment.

Next, apply a plastic covering over the soaked flannel cloth. On top of that place a heating pad and turn it up to the medium setting to begin with – then to high if the body tolerates it. Then perhaps it will help if you wrap a towel, folded lengthwise, around the entire area and fasten it with safety pins. The pack should remain in place between one and one-and-a-half hours.

The skin should be cleansed afterwards using a solution made with one quart of water and two teaspoons of baking soda. Use this to cleanse the abdomen. Store the flannel pack in a plastic container as it may be used for more than one application.

Frequency: 1›2›3›4›5›6›7 consecutive days per week.
Note: Take olive oil by mouth every third treatment, if directed, in amounts tolerated.

I also have great admiration for the work of Dr Virginia Livingston-Wheeler. Over the years I have attended quite a few of her lectures and we have taken part in seminars together.

After having finished medical school, her research showed that a microbe which she later named Progenitor Criptocides (PC) was present in all cancer cells. 'Progenitor' means that it has been on earth for millennia – in fact, forms that look like the microbe had been found in rock formed long before man appeared on earth. 'Criptocides' means 'the hidden killer'.

Although the microbe has been known before her research, no one had realised that its effect on the body could be the real cause of cancer.

Dr Livingston-Wheeler believes that the discovery was hard to track, because the disease itself advances in cycles, according to the form that PC takes at any one time.

In order to understand the way cancer cells reproduce, we need to know how normal cells function. When normal adult human cells need protein to repair tissue or when children need protein for growth and repair, they must get a pattern for that protein from the DNA in the nucleus of the cell. Once the pattern is made, the RNA in the cell manufactures as many of the proteins as the DNA orders. This manufacture of patterns works against us and in favour of viruses. It is known that viruses which contain DNA and RNA, or both, get into the body, enter a cell and transfer their pattern to the DNA or RNA of that cell. The cell automatically starts copying our molecule, according to that pattern. If the pattern is one for energy or for protein to make muscles, it reproduces that pattern. If it is for a virus, the cell produces viruses. The viruses spread all over the body and we have a viral disease.

Thus the cells received their pattern by mistake and continue to turn out more and more cells. If our immune system had been strong enough to destroy the PC microbe, these problems would not have arisen.

In order to prevent cancer, then, we need a healthy immune system which will destroy the PC. Nature indeed did provide for that, but man-made food which has much of the food value removed destroys the white blood cells and antibodies of the immune system, which should destroy the PC microbes.

Also, if we don't have enough nutrients (vitamins, minerals, proteins, carbohydrates, fats and water), we won't have the material with which to make the antibodies or the white blood cells, and thus we can't win the fight against cancer.

This is the reasoning behind the cancer therapy which is practised at the Livingston-Wheeler Clinic in San Diego, California.

Treatment at the clinic includes laetrile, enzymes, vitamins, minerals and dietary management.

The total commitment of people like Dr Virginia Livingston-Wheeler, Dr Hans Nieper, Drs Ernst Krebs, both father and son, Dr John A. Richardson and Dr Josef Issels, to name but a few, is remarkable and we owe them a great debt. They have been prepared to stand by their convictions and have risked ridicule for their unorthodox methods.

Dr William D. Kelley and I have discussed this commitment and drive to further research and knowledge several times. He originally qualified as a dentist and has studied non-toxic cancer therapy for a long time now.

In a previous chapter I have already praised him for his nutritional studies, but omitted to mention that he himself had cancer and failed to realise it for years. He said that he had experienced many of the true warning signs, which he ignored. We can profit from learning what he now believes were the warnings:

–gas on stomach or bowel;
–sudden weakness of the eyes;
–tired feeling most of the time;
–muscle weakness and cramps – first in the back and then in the chest;
–extreme mental depression;
–sudden change in hair texture and/or colour;
–development of various hernias (only in slow-growing tumours);
–confusion and difficulty in making even simple decisions.

All of these, says Dr Kelley, are signs of not being able to digest and assimilate proteins. He is of the opinion that a tumour is a sign of a deficiency of enzymes that digest protein. Thus meat is not allowed in his programme because all available enzymes are needed to digest the tumour itself. The sick body does not have enough enzymes to digest food protein, much less enzymes to digest the tumour. Since enzymes circulate in the blood, the ease of the cure depends on the amount of blood supplied to the cancer. An organ with a low blood supply, such as bone, recovers slowly. An organ with a high blood supply, such as lymph nodes, recovers more quickly, because more enzymes are available to digest the tumour.

Vitamins are important because they are co-enzymes. Even if enough enzymes do exist, they will not be able to function if the co-enzymes are not present. It is the same with minerals. They activate the enzyme/co-enzyme systems, and all three must be available in sufficient quantity.

Dr Kelley uses eight nutritional supplements:

1. a co-enzyme, vitamin, mineral compound;
2. a digestant;
3. a vitamin C complex;
4. organic minerals and trace elements;
5. almonds – these are eaten at exactly specified times and in exactly specified amounts;
6. amino acid supplements to assure the body a supply of protein that is easy to digest;
7. a pancreatic enzyme combination;
8. hydrochloric acid to digest proteins in the stomach.

With the combination of these supplements and the diet, the tumour begins to dissolve after a period ranging from three hours to 12 days. But the dissolving tumour can be toxic enough to kill the patient. The mass of the tumour must be dissolved and excreted through the blood stream very slowly, so that the circulation will not be overloaded. An overload causes toxicity in the body. The faster the toxins are released, the greater the strain on the system, and the more the danger of the patient succumbing to the toxins.

In his detoxification methods Dr Kelley usually recommends only one coffee enema a day for most patients – every morning, unless there is extreme toxicity, then another one is taken in the evening. The evening coffee enema could interfere with sleep and warm distilled water may be preferred. He does, however, point out that an extremely advanced case of cancer may need quite a few more enemas.

In his book *One Answer to Cancer*, Dr Kelley has described his detoxification therapy in great detail and has made it clear that patients are able to follow these guidelines in the privacy of their own home.

Another practitioner whom I admire greatly is Dr Ann Wigmore. She is a very dedicated lady and I have already mentioned her earlier in this book. According to her theories a vital force in the prevention and treatment of cancer seems to be wheatgrass extract. It is made from wheat, grown to a height of six to seven inches, cut close to the soil. It is then ground and mixed with an equal amount of water, and drunk daily.

Dr Wigmore heads the Hippocrates Health Institute at Boston and her doctrine embraces body, mind and spirit, i.e. she intends to deal with the whole person.

Her treatment includes diet, exercise, a positive mental outlook, self-discipline and a responsible attitude towards one's own health. During many years of study and tests, Dr Wigmore realised that wheatgrass has outstanding healing qualities; indeed the extract can be used for many ailments other than cancer.

The wheatgrass extract is combined with a completely vegetarian diet of raw live foods with plenty of raw fruit juice. She advocates enemas to detoxify the system and, initially, wheatgrass is also used for this purpose. Depending on the severity of the illness, patients remain at her clinic for three weeks or longer. The detoxification programme during the first few weeks is demanding, time consuming, and therefore best undertaken in the clinic. After the initial period the enemas can be eliminated but the patient continues to take wheatgrass cocktails and the live foods.

As I have already mentioned, the healing qualities of the wheatgrass extract are also used for other ailments. Tests are currently taking place to determine its possible curative effect on AIDS.

Dr Wigmore is a great believer in the principle that the responsibility for our own bodies rests with ourselves. I remember an official dinner during a conference to which Dr Wigmore declined the invitation. She claims that that is where it all starts! She is certainly a very principled and dedicated person.

The anthroposophical clinic in Switzerland is headed by Dr Rita Leroi and many cancer patients have received treatment there according to their unique approach.

The gentle approach of anthroposophy is harmonic

understanding of the human being in his or her mental, religious, scientific, cultural, physical and other expressions. The doctrine for the anthroposophical approach (based on the Greek word *anthropos*, meaning 'man') was founded by the Austrian scientist and philosopher Rudolf Steiner.

The theory is steadily receiving recognition all over the world, as it embraces prevention of illness and the promotion and restoration of health. Worldwide, many doctors trained in orthodox medicine have come to appreciate homoeopathy, herbal remedies and the anthroposophical approach, including therapies such as baths, massage, diet and, above all for cancer patients, the use of Iscador, as discussed in Chapter 7.

Cancer or leukaemia patients who have visited or stayed at the Swiss Ida Wegman's clinic have been guided physically and mentally.

I have immense respect for a colleague practitioner who still continues his work in helping to ease the human suffering, even though years ago he was given only a few months to live himself. He attended the Swiss clinic for treatment and now returns there once a year to keep his condition under control.

Dr Leroi monitors her patients with great responsibility and even after referring them to local practitioners she remains in touch and is always available to be called upon for advice.

It is sometimes interesting to look into the background and personal motivation of medical researchers and innovators. In this respect I must tell you about the origins of the Hoxsey Clinic. This medical centre started many years ago on the strength of an herbal tea mixture, an ointment and a powder, based on a recipe that had been in the Hoxsey family since the middle of the nineteenth century and handed down from father to son.

The story begins in 1840 at their ranch in Illinois. One of their prize horses had developed a noxious, spreading sore on its leg. The vet diagnosed it as cancer and said that the horse should be shot. John Hoxsey persuaded his father not to destroy the animal, but let nature take its course. It was then noticed that every morning the horse would head for the same part of the pasture and eat only herbs and plants that grew there. After a week or so the sore began to look better. It dried up, started to shrink and eventually began to separate from the surrounding tissue. After three months Hoxsey could slip a knife underneath and remove it. By the end of the year the horse's leg was completely healed.

Hoxsey reasoned that the cancer had regressed because of something in the plants which the horse had eaten. He picked each of the plants and mixed them in various combinations, trying them on other sick horses. He finally found three formulae to be effective most of the time: a liquid, a salve and a powder. News spread across the countryside and many farmers brought their ailing horses to the Hoxseys and many of them were cured. Only on his deathbed did Hoxsey pass on the secret formula to his son, who in turn passed it on to his son.

Eventually a medical clinic was opened in Dallas, Texas, and patients came from far afield. Many patients were willing to testify as to the effectiveness of the cure, but the medical establishment continually hounded Hoxsey and eventually forced him to close his clinic. In the 1960s he opened the Hoxsey Bio-Medical Center in Tijuana, Mexico, and still his patients come from all over the world and are willing to testify to remarkable recoveries.

In addition to the ointment and tea, treatment at the clinic includes herbs, vitamins, diet and interferon. They also use BCG (the TB vaccine), and live cell therapy (but not when the tumour is active). The injected cells from healthy young animals correspond to the cells in the patient's body that are damaged and have caused illness. The new cells travel in the blood to replace the damaged cells and help the patient to recover.

In contrast to the Hoxseys, my good friend Dr Serge Jurasunas has been more fortunate in his dealings with the medical establishment in Portugal.

I have visited him several times in his lovely clinic there, where he has a very busy practice. A while ago the Portuguese medical authorities expressed their recognition of his work in the opening of a new wing to a hospital and inviting Dr Jurasunas to practise alternative medicine there. In doing so, patients are now at liberty to choose either orthodox or alternative therapies, or a combination of the two.

I strongly believe that this choice should be available worldwide and hope to see this example followed by medical authorities elsewhere.

For your information I reproduce below the metabolic programme designed and adhered to by Dr Jurasumas, which has proved sufficiently successful for it to be introduced in clinics in other countries as well. I admit that it may appear confusing and complicated at first glance, but patients have shown a remarkably positive response to the programme. More detailed instructions and information on the various components of the programme are also given.

Daily metabolic programme:
One hour before breakfast:
One herb enema made from essential oil and clay (important to wash out the bowels and remove waste matter and toxins).
Thirty minutes before breakfast:
One glass of detoxification drink to aid the disposal of mucous from the bowels.
With breakfast:
Two capsules of germanium (or more if necessary).
Two 500 mg tablets of vitamin C.
Middle of the morning:
Take a hot osmotic enzyme herb bath for 20 minutes. During the bath, take one ampoule of Apizellin.
Thirty minutes before lunch:
Two ampoules of Apizellin;
L39 – 45 drops in a half-cup of water together with a cup of detoxification drink.
Lunch:
One ampoule of Apiaprophican liquid;

Two capsules of germanium.
One hour before dinner:
A coffee enema.
Thirty minutes before dinner:
One cup of detoxification drink.
Dinner:
Two to four germanium capsules;
D.O.M. n° 3-4 – one capsule of each;
Two 500 mg tablets of vitamin C.
Before going to bed:
One ampoule of Apiaprophican liquid;
L39 – 45 drops;
One cup of Pau d'Arco.

Further instructions and information
Herb enema:
For one litre of water use:
> 1 tablespoon of rosemary
> 1 tablespoon of lavender
> 1 tablespoon of basil
> 3 drops of essence of eucalyptus
> 1 tablespoon of powder clay
> ½ teaspoon of powdered thyme
> 1 head of garlic

Bring to the boil, let cool and strain.

Coffee enema:
Three heaped tablespoons of grounded roast coffee beans to one litre of water. Bring to the boil and simmer for 20 minutes. Cool and strain.

DOM (Detoxification Organic Metabolism)
These capsules are made from herbs to help detoxification of the blood, liver, kidneys and bowels. They also contain enzymes. DOM is very important to help the body to support the high toxicity due to the breakdown of the tumour.

134

The capsules contain herbs such as yellow dock, echinacea, marigold, liquorice, chelidonium, Ipe Roxo, comfrey root, sarsaparilla root etc.

In certain cases a mixture of essential-oil herbs is also given in drops which are very powerful and, as well as their immunological factor, will stimulate the oxido-reduction of the blood. Aromavit, made from seven essential-oil herbs, is used.

Detoxification drink:
The preparation of linseed juice, used in this drink, requires two tablespoons of linseed for two litres of water. Simmer for 40 minutes. Cool and store in a refrigerator.

The detoxification drink can be made from the following ingredients:
    ½ cup of linseed juice
    ½ cup of pineapple juice
    ½ cup of carrot juice
    1 tablespoon of liquid chlorophyll
    ½ cup of distilled water

Pau d'Arco (Ipe Roxo):
This is a herb from the bark of a tree which has been used in various forms over a number of years. It can be prepared as a tea, but can also be taken in stronger dosages as a tonic. It is recommended in cases of tumours or leukaemia. Pau d'Arco tablets are of cytotastic value in cancer cases.

Increasing immunity:
Building up the immune system, as we have learned, is very important. Several substances and vitamins are recommended to this end:
    –ginseng
    –zinc
    –magnesium
    –vitamin C
    –vitamin B group

Apizellin ampoules contain high dosage of ginseng, zinc, magnesium, etc.

Apiaprophican liquid also contains methionin to protect the liver, and yeast is obtained from the vitamin B group.

Germanium will stimulate the production of interferon in the body.

The L39 drops contain ingredients to detoxicate the body and to increase the immune system. Similar to the co-enzyme as a famous catalyser for the immune system.

Sulphur and Pulsatilla will stimulate the elimination of toxic substances.

Osmotic herb bath:
Half fill the bathtub with water at a temperature of about 103° F. Dissolve in this a mixture of herbs together with essential oils. Then fill up the bath, raising the temperature to 110° F.

After bathing, rinse the herbs off the body.

Wrap up in a blanket to keep the body warm while relaxing.

Make a muddy paste with the herbs, using six tablespoons of herbs, mixed with water, to make a layer 8 cm square and place this over the liver area. Cover with a cloth.

A hot pack should be applied to heat these herbs and help penetration through the skin.

Last but not least, I conclude with the Bristol Clinic in our own country. This alternative health centre provides a complementary approach to cancer, aimed, yet again, at treating the whole person. The clinic was opened in July 1983 by HRH the Prince of Wales and he signed the visitors' book.

Several of the different methods and ideas mentioned in this chapter are used in this clinic. In addition, Dr Alec Forbes, founder member of the Bristol Clinic, has introduced several of his own.

Let us be grateful that, slowly but surely, the message is coming across that people who suffer these dreadful diseases deserve all the help we can give them. Mind control, autogenic training, mental exercises are all taught to patients at the

136

Bristol Clinic, in order to stimulate their ability to beat cancer.

One of my co-lecturers, Dr Ian Pearce, recognised the need for cancer patients to have emotional support. As an orthodox doctor he found that much more could be done in that direction. In his lectures he supported a sensible approach to cancer and instructed patients that they are responsible mentally and physically for their own health. It is now widely recognised that counselling plays an important role in the guidance of patients.

Patients at the Bristol Clinic benefit from the ideas of Dr Pearce. An open letter he wrote to his colleagues serves as the preface to the book *New Approaches to Cancer*, written by the very able Shirley Harrison. It states that doctors today hold the key to every front door in the country in numerous opportunities we find in new techniques and therapies, all a vita part in the healing or prevention of cancer.

In this chapter I have tried to deal with several of the many treatment methods used worldwide. Many practitioners have discussed and lectured on their respective theories and from all of them we have been able to learn something. If we are not prepared or willing to learn any more, it points to a closed mind and poorer person as a result. With such an attitude we can achieve very little, especially when it comes to medical problems as influential as those discussed in this book.

If, in summing up, we analyse all the different therapies, we find that in principle the goal is everywhere the same. The methods differ in execution, but they all seem to have one view in mind and that is to help reduce human suffering, to heal and to prevent.

All over the world responsible practitioners and researchers are at work. The goal everywhere is the same. How can we best help people who suffer?

We all recognise the needs for a sensible diet, building up the body, dissolving the tumour, eliminating the waste products, fighting degenerative cells and helping people towards better health.

The responsibility is ours, patients and practitioners alike. We have to combine body, mind and spirit to fight the most feared disease of all time – cancer.

For nearly a century, scientists worldwide have studied thousands of compounds in search of the ultimate benefit. Finally, one researcher has discovered the breakthrough that many have been hoping for – a nutritional formula that greatly increases natural killer cell activity. Enzymatic Theraphy's Cell Forte IP-6 is the unique combination of inositol and inositol hexaphosphate (IP-6), researched and patented by Dr A. Shamsuddin MD, PhD.

Cell Forte IP-6
Enhances Natural Cellular Defences
Virtually all of our bodies' cells contain and require IP-6 for healthy function. Cell Forte boosts our natural cellular defences by increasing the levels of inositol phosphates in our cells. This heightened activity strengthens our cells and entire immune system helping to kill abnormal molecules that could otherwise damage cells.

What is IP-6?
It is a natural compound found primarily in grains and soybeans. The IP-6 Cell Forte comes from the bran portion of brown rice. Rice is a staple for most Asian diets. This may help explain why they have fewer health problems often accociated with our westernised, low-fibre diet.

More Effective Together
Scientists have long known about the individual health benefits of both inositol and inositol hexaphosphate. But Dr Shamsuddin had the vision to show these two compounds are more effective working together than individually. The conslusion: after 15 years of scientific study, Cell Forte IP-6 has proven to be a monumental breakthrough – a safe, one-of-a-kind product with uniquely powerful health benefits.

10

Visualisation and Outlook

WHEN I WAS YOUNGER our neighbours had a daughter who was terminally ill. Her parents had made up her bed in front of the window so that she was able to look out and see what was going on outside. Everyone passing by would wave to her. She spent a lot of time there, as the deterioration process was slow and I often popped in for a chat with her. One day when I visited her she looked at the tree outside the window and said: "You know, Jan, when the last leaf of that tree comes down, I won't be here anymore."

Her parents heard the story, which obviously upset them and her father hit on the idea of painting a leaf, similar to the others, and planting this on the tree. While she was asleep one night he quietly made his way out to the tree and placed the artificial leaf where she would be able to see it.

She actually lived for quite a while after that, perhaps wondering why that leaf had not fallen. Although she continued to deteriorate, there was still some quality to her life and she still took pleasure in watching others get on with their lives. Her parents made her as comfortable as possible, but the day eventually came when we had to say goodbye to her and she died peacefully.

The thought behind this story is that a positive outlook and a determined frame of mind influences life and, moreover, improves the quality of it. I often think back to one particular lecture I attended on cancer. It was given by a French professor and the lecture was followed by a question and answer session. I remember one of my colleagues asking an unusual question and the professor responded by asking why she would want to pose that particular one.

She then replied that she herself had cancer. Immediately the professor reacted: "Please do not ever use the word cancer again. When you put it like that, you influence yourself negatively and make your problems worse."

That was a lesson, because whatever we do in life, if we approach it negatively, we will get a negative response. If it is approached positively the response will be positive.

The theory behind visualisation techniques is that positive thinking will help us get through certain critical times in our life, and for many cancer patients it can serve as a transition into another stage, where sometimes improvement can be realised.

One of my patients had been involved in the Windscale disaster. Although he did not in fact have cancer, after the disaster his health had broken down. We had lengthy discussions, during which I realised that his confidence had been badly shaken, which adversely affected his health. Immediately after the disaster he had resigned from the plant and looked for other work. During our conversations he began to discover himself and his values and set out to rebuild his shattered career and confidence by determining his motivations. His positive action resulted in regained health and he could once more enjoy a good quality of life. Whatever we do, we should always heed the warnings and positively consider what we are doing.

I remember one occasion when I was returning to Scotland by air after a visit to London. As I was boarding the plane I recognised a stewardess as being a patient of mine. She asked me if I would like to visit the cockpit during the flight and, of course, I accepted this offer gratefully.

Sitting in the cockpit, enjoying the magnificent view, I was fascinated by the complexity of the control panels. Only to the pilot and navigator would all these knobs and lights make any sense. The only two signs I could relate to were "Caution" and "Danger". As far as I was concerned these two warnings signified whether or not we were to land safely at our destination.

The friendly pilot tried to explain some of the procedure before landing and expressed his appreciation of the fact that the runway was clearly visible when we came into land at Glasgow Airport. I remember how well laid out and lit up it was. Although he would have been able to land with his instruments, this pilot was no exception in his profession by preferring to see what he was doing. Clear vision gave him that extra confidence.

After we landed safely, I asked him if he ever gave a thought to the people whose lives were in his hands or whether his time in the cockpit just meant flying time to him. He chuckled and answered that that factor of his work was more taxing mentally than any other aspect.

I could not help but compare the control panels in the cockpit to the human body. In the latter case, if anything goes wrong no warning lights flash on and off, but niggling aches and pains develop which are a sure sign that somewhere something is amiss. If we then have a clear vision, we will know that something ought to be done. Like the pilot flying on his instruments, we can survive for a period of time, but the pilot can always rely on ground control and his instruments. If we disregard the warning signs what have we to fall back on?

Many illnesses and diseases are brought upon ourselves through carelessness or insufficient attention to our way of life. Possibly twenty years ago I would have hesitated before saying this, but now I am completely convinced that some of the causes of cancer are related to what we eat and drink and how we lead our lives.

We need always to keep our vision clear and visualise the beauty of nature and its remarkable innate powers that enable us to maintain our health. Even when we are struck by illness or disease, let us then be positive and remember that nature is the greatest healer!

In front of me I have a letter written by the mother of a teenager who was a cancer patient. The girl had been diagnosed as suffering from progressive cancer in the bones. The mother and her husband recognised their responsibility as parents and did everything possible to encourage their daughter into believing in complete recovery. The thinking of both parents and the daughter centred on this and they visualised and planned for a life after recovery — and the girl did indeed recover. In her letter the mother enclosed a photograph of their daughter, now a member of an orchestra, visiting Switzerland on a concert tour. The girl looks happy and well and, to me, symbolises the transformation possible through positive thinking.

Of course, recovery cannot always be the outcome and whether it is or not is certainly not our decision. But even when things go wrong, it must be a comfort to know that one has done everything possible. Isn't that so much better than accepting the irresponsible attitude exemplified by: "I have a problem and I have to learn to live with it!"

In this context I have great admiration for the parents of young twins, when it became apparent that one of the little ones had a brain tumour. I admired the parents for not leaving a single stone unturned in their search to improve the little girl's condition. They showed great faith and this seemed to be reflected in the fight the young girl put up. The specialists and surgeons could hardly believe her struggles, because they thought that she should have expired long before. In the end, unfortunately, the little girl did die. Nevertheless, some comfort could be gained from the fact that everything possible had been attempted and at no time had the parents given up hope.

The mystery of life is in the hands of our Creator, who gives life and takes life. Despite that, we are obliged to act responsibly with His great gift of life.

Just a few weeks ago I again saw a lady who had been a cancer patient about fourteen years ago. When she came to me at that time she had been in a very poor physical condition, but of determined spirit. After she had undergone treatment for a while she regained her health, which enabled her to return to her work as a missionary and her life was certainly a blessing for many others. That is what I call good vision — to be able to translate gratitude for life and health into trying to help others. How often are we not guilty of giving in? That is the easy way out. Letting tensions and worries keep us from enjoying life to the full, will only serve to increase our problems.

The other day a lady who had undergone an operation for a mastectomy told me that she now felt well, but she knew that if she worried she would feel worse again. She had made up her mind not to look back any longer, but to look forward with the firm conviction that it would never happen again. That is the right attitude for cancer patients or for leukaemia patients. Always look forward to improvement.

There is no point in dishing out false hope to people or keeping them from facing reality. That would not be right either. Being realistic, however, does not need to exclude a positive outlook. We then stand a better chance of recovery, in which nature will be our ally.

Some patients are emotionally better equipped to deal with such traumatic issues and sometimes it is of great help if they can discuss their fears and expectations.

Recently I saw a young man who had just read a report published in 1986 estimating that more than 900,000 Americans will be diagnosed as suffering from cancer and about half of these people will die as a result within five years. He said of this: "I do not want to be on the losing side. I intend to be on the side of those who recover." That attitude is the best visualisation possible.

In this instance I would like to mention Dr Ray Evers, who

has spent a lifetime researching degenerative diseases. Where he could have chosen to lead a relatively uncomplicated life by restricting his medical commitment to practising as a general practitioner, he elected to serve mankind to the best of his abilities. He has been under threat of imprisonment on account of his unorthodox convictions. Yet his message has remained clear: *If it is to be, it is up to me.*

It is our responsibility to work out how we can fight and conquer our problems. We need only look over Dr Ray Evers' long list of case histories and testimonials to know that his quote contains much wisdom and that a positive attitude is what he aims to instil in his patients.

The kind of treatment is perhaps of secondary importance, if only we approach that treatment with a positive attitude, a positive mind and with a vision of improvement in the future.

A continental doctor visited me not so long ago and wondered how it was possible that during clinical trials with laetrile, one patient was considered to be cured while others had not responded to the same extent. That patient was lucky that laetrile had proved effective in his case, because often much more is required, such as dietary help, supplements and general guidance. However, he had continuously maintained a positive attitude and a fervent belief in recovery. This could well be the secret to improvement and in my mind most certainly also contributes to prevention.

A youngish woman had come to me in despair when she had been told that she had but little time to live. She told me: "I can't bear to think about it anymore, because I cannot cope and therefore I have taken up music again. Maybe it will divert my attention from my health problems." She did indeed find great solace in her music. She lived longer than had been anticipated, and for those few years left to her she lived happily. The sound of her music soothed the mental and emotional wounds created by cancer.

A wonderful visualisation therapy has been put together by Carl Simonton, a radiation oncologist, and by his wife, Stephanie Matthews Simonton, a psychotherapist. This

144

therapy has been designed with a view to good health and many patients have benefited from it. In dealing with cancer patients, Simonton saw clearly what visualisation could amount to and expressed this in several methods, one of which is described at the close of this chapter.

Patients often see cancer or a tumour as a localised problem, akin to a foreign object which must be got rid of as soon as possible. In this they will be facilitated by the Simonton approach. It works along similar lines to programming a computer: feed in the correct information and the computer will work out the problem. In the Simonton approach it is a matter of preparing the mind to stimulate physical functions. If fed the right information this will encourage the healthy cells to become stronger and more resilient.

Carl Simonton has said that cancer management today is in a state of confusion. It looks almost like the disease itself — fragmented and confused. Once we face up to the reality of the problem, we can then with a positive mind form a mental picture of a healthy cell, dividing and multiplying. From there we can continue trying to overcome feelings of despair, hopelessness, helplessness and darkness. It has been seen that the psychological effects of visualisation techniques can sometimes change our situations drastically.

The Simontons clearly recognised that cancer is not just a physical problem, but a problem affecting the whole person, so it includes the mind. Therefore strengthening the immune system by way of relaxation and visualisation techniques is an important aspect of treatment for cancer patients.

Even when dealing with death, visualisation therapy can be of great help and comfort in those difficult hours. The confrontation with death can be harsh for cancer patients, because of the often gradual drawn-out deterioration they have experienced. This is equally the case for their relatives and friends, as they feel so totally helpless and often can only stand by and witness the terminal process take place.

However, I have seen patients who were so much in control

145

as a result of visualisation techniques, that they were able to comfort and console the family in the final stages of their life.

In this category falls a family friend who had a great influence on me when I was growing up. I can only be grateful for having had a chance to know him so well during my formative years. Although we lost him when he was only thirty-eight years old, he greatly affected my future outlook on life. Death for him was unavoidable as in those days there were no effective treatments for leukaemia. He accepted his fate and concentrated on living while there still was life, accepting in a dignified manner that life for him would be short. He was of great comfort to those he was going to leave behind and I remember that shortly before he left us he spoke to me and said: "I am happy. Why are you not?" His vision was clearly directed to the future. In the knowledge that he had attempted everything possible, he accepted that there was nothing left to do but to say his farewells. That is the outlook we should all desire to have when death is unavoidable.

Is that what is so touching in the book written by Elisabeth Kübler-Ross, *To Live Until We Say Goodbye*? In this book she tells us how we can learn to accept the unavoidable, and relates some of the different traumas she has experienced with patients. She was able to teach them that there was nothing to fear.

In the foreword of her book it is said that the choice is always ours. When we have cancer we can naturally put our head in the sand and temporarily forget it. We can drown ourselves in self-pity, anger or anguish until it is too late. Or we can get the best possible help available to us in this country or abroad. It is that vision which made my friend say: "I am happy. Why are you not?" We should learn to give happiness a chance, even in the most terrible circumstances.

None of us can walk in clouds of happiness without ever facing reality. That is impossible. But I consider it a wonderful comfort to follow the advice of our Creator: "Be still and know that I am God."

In all our suffering and weakness, when understanding

146

and sympathy is needed, we can feel His presence, if we just let ourselves.

In the foreword to this book Dr Contreras mentioned the greatest physician of all times — Jesus of Nazareth, who showed the greatest love ever manifested on earth. He is Love and He is always beside us. If we can keep our vision on that great healer, we will get the help we need in the most difficult moments of our life.

In a letter I received from a lady, she explained that when one falls and breaks a bone, the falling is bad enough in that it results in a physical injury, but the mental injury of the fall takes much longer to heal. Physical healing can take place, but mental healing is equally important, as it will influence the physical healing process. Sometimes the fear of something to come is more debilitating than the actual occurrence. Consider for one minute a fresh wound. Immediately thousands of cells come into action and start the healing process and probably in a little while the wound will be healed.

Nature is remarkable in that millions of repair cells are available, intelligent and responsive to our thoughts: if we influence our cells positively towards any healing process, an enormous army of cells sets to work to heal the body with the great power that God has bestowed on us.

Responding to even minor vibrations, our body cells possess an innate intelligence enabling them to follow our directions. If we therefore look at perfect images and are imaginative in rebuilding the creative energy, a higher level of improvement can be achieved.

These vibrations can be thoughts or actions, and will result in reactions. Perhaps we can now understand how a positive mental and emotional attitude can readily help us to a manifestation of good health and strength. We can then also understand that the healing of disease by love and happiness are positive elements which will be victorious over emotions like fear, worry, hate, anxiety, envy, stress or any other destructive vibrations.

147

Since I began to instruct patients in visualisation or relaxation techniques, I have seen many cases which proved their effectiveness. I am strongly of the opinion, as a result of years of experience, that cancer can be overcome as well as prevented by establishing the right positive attitudes.

Sometimes a misconception first needs to be cleared away. There was the lady who asked me: "How can a dead cell come back to life once it is dead?" I had to inform her that once a cell has died, it will remain dead, because it cannot be reanimated. Even God will not bring a dead cell back to life. Yet, a dead cell or a carcinomic cell can be disposed of and be replaced by a new cell. Let us just consider that every six months in an adult life the cells are replaced. If a cell stays in the body for longer than this it can more readily become a carcinomic cell.

So we come back to the importance of dietary management in cancer treatment or prevention. It is to our advantage to use the life force within the food we eat for the renewal of cells. It is unfortunate that, mostly, people are unwilling to change their eating habits unless they become aware of medical complications. Often common sense does not prevail till then. It seems to present less of a problem for people to change their religion, their political views, their husband or wife! I have seen how difficult it is for most to change their eating habits.

A change in dietary management is unlikely to produce immediate results. After all, the problem did not spring up overnight. Be optimistic and never give in to say: "I am going to die", or "I will never get better". Instead reprogramme the mind with: "I am basically healthy and therefore I will be victorious over my problems". Always remember that without our life force we are lost.

In her book *Say NO To Cancer*, Barbara Waters puts forward an opinion that is worth considering: "Cancer is a disease of a body out of control. The state of balance and harmony are gone." She also writes: "Cancer cannot grow where there is a balanced metabolism in the body." These opinions signify direct knowledge and experience of the problem.

There is a cause for every effect and in this book we have

looked at causes, curative methods and prevention. Physical nourishment is most important. God inspired King Solomon to write: "Better to eat vegetables with people you love, than to eat the finest meat where there is hate" (Proverbs Ch. 15, v. 17; New Translation). This means that a mental attitude with no anxious thought for tomorrow, but faith in God through prayer and meditation, will cultivate the right thoughts of love, faith and joy.

King Solomon also wrote: "Being cheerful keeps you healthy. It is slow death to be gloomy all the time" (Proverbs Ch. 17, v. 22; New Translation).

The old naturopathic views on the beneficial effects of sunshine, fresh air and exercise are thankfully back in focus today. Healthy breathing will indeed help the vital process in the body which depends on oxygen. Take exercise in the fresh air wherever possible as this is always advantageous.

Do not be easily discouraged, because it is essential to understand that we have to be wholehearted in our efforts. The heart is the only organ that can never be attacked by cancer.

Let us meditate on the thought that if our heart is full of love, how much love we will then receive as a healing factor. This is the meaning of the visualisation or autogenic techniques, or any other positive-attitude techniques that will help us to overcome our troubles.

In front of me is a letter from a patient who was formerly in great despair. With some of the techniques I advised her of she has managed to lift herself up. When she got back home to her own country, she wrote to me that she felt deeply indebted for the care she had been shown, but also for the helping lift out of "a valley of misery".

I would like to end this book with a few guidelines for some of these simple techniques, although there are dozens of examples that can easily be obtained from a variety of organisations or books on the subject.

The first of these is a very worthwhile bone-breathing visualisation programme. The Chinese believe that the centre

149

of your bones are responsible for the well-being of the body as a whole. This exercise in visualisation, together with the relaxation that goes with it, is widely used for therapy for those with bone disorders.

You will use your breath by imagining the breath entering up and through the bones as you breathe in and, as you breathe out, it is passed down and away through the same path.

The first thing is to get yourself into a comfortable position either:

1. in the sitting position, in a comfortable upright chair, feet placed evenly on the floor, hands resting in the lap, spine straight, and the head resting comfortably, the top of the head in line with the ceiling; or
2. lying down on a comfortable mat, with the spine straight, arms to the side with the palms turned upwards, feet just a little way apart.

Begin to become aware of your breathing. Slow the breath right down, getting it as slow and deep as you can. Feel the breath right down into the bottom of the ribcage as you breathe in deep, slow, even breaths.

Begin to feel the body relaxing as you just concentrate your mind on the breath as it comes in and out, relaxing and letting go.

Now imagine your body:

1. Imagine the breath coming in and through the bones of the left foot, up the bones of the leg to the hip bone. Then, as you breathe out, the breath returns the same way and out through the left foot. Repeat seven times.
2. Then imagine the breath coming in and up through the bones of the right foot, up the bones of the leg to the hip and then, as you breathe out, the breath returns the same way and out through the right foot. Repeat seven times.

3.   Now breathe in through the bones of the left foot up the left leg, cross through the pelvis and, as you breathe out, send the breath down the bones and out through the right foot. Repeat seven times.

4.   Now breathe in and up through bones of the left hand, up through the bones of the left arm to the shoulder. Breathe out and return down and out the same way. Repeat seven times.

5.   Now breathe in and up through the bones of the right hand and up the right arm, to the shoulder. Then breathe out and down the same way. Repeat seven times.

6.   Breathe in and take breath in through the left arm, across from left shoulder to right shoulder, then breathing out down the right arm and out through the bones of the right hand. Breathe in and up to the left shoulder and breathe out down the left arm and out through the left hand. Repeat seven times.

7.   Breathing in, take the breath up the spine to the top, and then, as you breathe out, send the breath down the spine again and out through the base. Repeat seven times.

8.   Imagine the skull. Take a breath in and direct it up and over the head to the front, breathing out. Take the breath out through the skull and back. Repeat seven times.

9.   Now imagine the body as a whole. Take the breath in, up from both feet and up through all the bones in the body to the top of the head, breathing down and out through all the bones and out through the feet. Repeat seven times.

It may be easier to visualise the breath in terms of a colour, or a light or a feeling of warmth, whatever you find the easiest, and repeat the whole exercise as often as you like. It may seem a little difficult at first, especially if this is the first time you have done any visualisation, but persevere and soon it will flow and you will receive great benefit.

I will now set down some of the principles of the Simonton meditation as they have been explained by the Simontons in their books and workshops.

After having relaxed along the lines I have explained when talking about the bone breathing visualisation, follow the instructions below.

Imagine that you see your cancer cells. Try to make as clear a picture of them as you can. Perhaps you belong to those people who can visualise very easily. Then just skip the next sentences. Or perhaps you belong to those people who do not see anything when closing their eyes. Then you are most likely an auditive person and you just tell yourself the story that the better visualisers are seeing with their mind's eye. Both ways are equally good and give the same results.

Now in visualising the cancer cells, see them as they really are: sickly, weak cells, more bone than flesh, whose only power lies in hiding from the immune system, but who cannot really fight back. And now imagine strong, powerful, purposeful white bloodcells. They come right on, like soldiers on the march.

Perhaps at the same time the body is being treated with X-rays. Then see how each X-ray is a dart, mortally wounding the cancer cells, but only irritating the strong white cells, so that they attack with more vigour. Or perhaps the body is being treated with chemotherapy. Then see the sickly cells avidly drinking the poison and dying, but see how the white cells are far too smart to do that. See how they consume large quantities of the good vitamins and minerals you are feeding them. Now see how they attack the sickly cells. They are just devouring them. They are dumping the debris in the circulation and it will be taken out of the body.

Some people are not able to see cells. They have no imagination for such things. Never mind. If you see your cancer cells as little gnawing mice, like animals, and your white cells as big, strong cats eating those mice, or if you see

152

the cancer cells as weak, malformed little fish and your white cells as sharks devouring them, it is all right. You are allowed to make the picture that suits you best as long as you picture your cancer cells as few, sickly and weak and your white bloodcells as strong, vigorous and victorious.

The aim is to build a new computer programme in your brain, changing the cancer growth into cancer control. Building such a new programme costs time and endurance. You must not look at lumps in your body and wonder if perhaps they are shrinking already, but aim to change the messages from the brain to the body.

You should do such an exercise three times a day. Then when you have finished your meditation, call the strength slowly back into your relaxed muscles, pat yourself on the back for a job well done and that is it.

Sometimes people interpose something else between relaxation and visualisation and also between visualisation and taking back their strength. And that is going, in your mind, to a place you like very much. See yourself in a beautiful park, under a particularly lovely tree, or somewhere in the mountains, or perhaps at the side of a lake. Just choose a place you like very much and study everything around you. Hear the birds, breathe the fresh air, feel and smell the grass. Make all your senses participate in this exercise. It is a good preparation for the visualisation, and a good in-between-land to return to after your battle with the cancer cells.

There are some people who have compassion even towards their cancer cells. They are appalled by this talk of battle and war, about eating and devouring, killing and destroying. Do not despair — for them there is another exercise, which they may devise themselves. It is about sickly cancer cells, and kind, big teaching cells coming along. Taking them one by one to a nice, warm place and teaching them how to behave. Just as delinquent children often can be turned into useful members of society, merely by taking them out of their slums and giving them a good wholesome diet, it has been proved that cancer cells can be turned back into normal ones. So, if

153

you feel you do not belong to the warriors of the world, this is a gentle programme that perhaps has more appeal to you and that can be used as successfully as the more aggressive programme.

Do this exercise three times daily. Make sure you cannot be interrupted during this period. Take fifteen to twenty minutes each time, because the steady drop hollows the stone!

It is my sincere wish that this book be of help and guidance to cancer patients and their relations. Let it also point a way to prevention of cancer and leukaemia. Do something about it today. Bear in mind the old Sanskrit saying:

"Yesterday is but a dream, tomorrow is but a vision. But today well-lived makes every yesterday a dream of happiness and every tomorrow a vision of hope. Look well therefore to this day."

Bibliography and Literature

A. Vogel — *Krebs* — *Schiksal oder Zivilisations Krankheit*, Verlag A. Vogel, Teufen, Switzerland.

Shirley Harrison — *New Approaches to Cancer*, Century Hutchinson Ltd., London.

Ross Horne — *The Health Revolution*, Ross Horne, Avalon Beach, NSW, Australia.

Virginia Livingston-Wheeler, MD — *The Microbiology of Cancer*, The Livingston-Wheeler Medical Publications, USA.

Richard Ericson, BS, JD — *Cancer Treatment* — *Why So Many Failures?*, G.E.P.S., Cancer Memorial Publisher, Illinois, USA.

Ewan Cameron and Linus Pauling — *Cancer and Vitamin C*, The Linus Pauling Institute of Science and Medicine, USA.

Roderich Menzel — *Ongeneeslijke Ziekte te Genezen?*, U.M. West Friesland, Hoorn, the Netherlands.

Ralph R. Hovananian — *Medical Dark Ages*, Ralph R. Hovnanian, 2128 Prospect Ave., Evanston, USA.

Susan G. Cole — *The Patient's Guide to Cancer Care*, Health Improvements Research Corp., New York, USA.

Brenda Kidman — *A Gentle Way with Cancer*, Century Arrow, London.

Ross Trattler — *Better Health through Natural Healing*, Thorson Publishing Group, Wellingborough, Northants.

155

Deepak Chopra, MD — *Creating Health*, Houghton Mifflin Co., Boston, USA.

Barbara Waters, — *Say NO to Cancer*, Nutritional Therapy, Scottsdale, New Zealand.

Charles F. Haanel — *The Master Key*, R. and W. Heap Publishing Co., London.

J. D. Tossaint, MD — *Ziekte Als Lot en Kans*, Ankh-Hermes BV, Deventer, the Netherlands.

Fritjof Capra — *The Turning Point*, Flamingo, published by Fontana Paperbacks, London.

Elisabeth Kübler-Ross — *To Live Until We Say Goodbye*, Prentice-Hall Inc., Englewood Cliffs, NJ, USA.

Ruth Yale Long, PhD — *Crackdown on Cancer with Good Nutrition*, Nutrition Education Ass. Inc., Texas, USA.

O. Carl Simonton, Stephanie Matthews-Simonton and James Creighton — *Getting Well Again*, J. P. Tarche, Inc., 1978.

H. C. Moolenburgh — *Fluoride: The Freedom Fight*, Mainstream Publishing, Edinburgh.

Index

157